Super Kid

Super Kid

Super Smart
Newton? Mozart? Rembrandt?

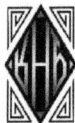

By Neuro Geeks

SUPER KID
SUPER SMART
BY NEURO GREEKS
***

All material contained herein is Copyright
Copyright © Neuro Geeks 2022
***

Paperback ISBN: 979-8-9869299-4-1
ePub ISBN: 979-8-2153750-2-0
***

Written by Neuro Geeks
Published by Royal Hawaiian Press
Cover art by Tyrone Roshantha
Publishing Assistance by Dorota Reszke
***

For more works by this author, please visit:
www.royalhawaiianpress.com
***

Table of Contents

1.1 Welcome

You're about to embark on the neuroscience program for parents. We have so much amazing information to share with you. So why neuroscience for parents? Well, obviously your child has a brain and brain science in general has seen a tremendous development over the last 10 years. We've never known so much about the brain and yet this is still the beginning. New insights into how our brain is functioning are discovered every year and it's pretty safe to say that neuroscience nowadays is one of the most exciting scientific fields of our time.

The brain of your child is amazing. It records everything. It's formatted through its interaction with its environment and those experiences. From the very first moments they are born until adolescence, it will heavily impact who they will become as an adult, and how they will interact with others. It determines how they will love and trust others, how they will react to authority and power, how they will overcome adversity or not and in general, how successful they're going to be later in life.

There was a study done over three decades in Minnesota. They measured and analyzed all kinds of things. And one of the most confronting findings was that the researchers were able to predict with 77 percent accuracy if a student would drop out of high school and this only by looking at the quality of care given when he or she was only three and a half years old.

So yes, we as parents have a huge responsibility in the development of our children. It's actually a double responsibility when you think of it. First, we as parents were responsible for 50 percent of the gene pool of our kids and our partner makes up for the other 50 percent. Now on top of that, these kids and their genes will interact with their environment which will trigger these genes to activate or not. This environment of course is one where we as a parent again constitute the vast majority of influence.

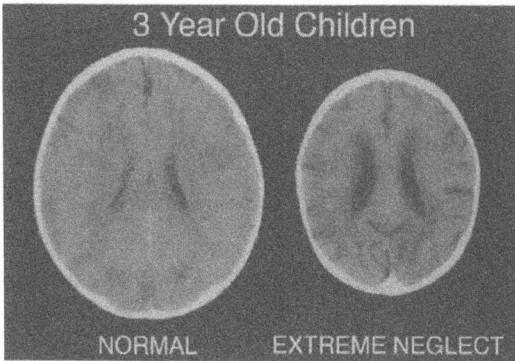

These images illustrate the negative impact of neglect on the developing brain. The CT scan on the left is from a healthy three-year-old with an average head size. The image on the right is from a three year old child suffering from severe sensory-deprivation neglect. This child's brain is significantly smaller and has abnormal development of cortex.

How we treat our children affects their brain development. Now this image is an extreme case of this. Here we see two brain scans of two three-year-old and the one on the left had a normal environment and upbringing. Now the one on the right on the other hand was facing extreme neglect. And yes, it is as bad as it looks. Now don't worry. This is an extreme case.

If you're angry at your kid once and end up yelling, give him or her a slap on the wrist, that won't result in this extreme cortical atrophy as you can see here. I just wanted to show you this image as an extreme proof that we as parents have a real impact on our children's brain development. Funny enough, the opposite is true as well.

Becoming a parent has a huge impact on the parent's brain as well. The most dramatic is the impact on neurogenesis. Neurogenesis is the creation of new brain cells. Parents turn out are subject to so much stress due to their offspring directly or indirectly, that this significantly lowers their neurogenesis when compared to adults who don't have kids. Now, in recent years we've become more aware of the importance of adult neurogenesis in keeping a healthy brain.

This actually is already measurable in the brain of pregnant women. Imagine that the brain of pregnant women physically shrinks during pregnancy. Now, before some of you start to make some lame jokes about this, after delivery their brain goes back to its normal size. Another way that parents' brain is impacted is through the release of oxytocin and its effects.

It was Professor Walter Freeman at Berkeley who found that there was a massive reorganization of our brain cells when we first started parenting. You probably have heard about oxytocin, right? It's called the bonding hormone or the love hormone. In women. Oxytocin is released during labor and breastfeeding and that makes of course a lot of sense as it helps the mother to bond with her newborn child.

But that's not the only role of the oxytocin and vasopressin, its male counterpart. plays. When we become a parent and we're all overwhelmed with love and awe, and we hold that little baby, and we do the stuff young parents do, well that's when we release oxytocin and vasopressin. The effect of these hormones helps us to bond with the baby of course. But it goes further than that.

These hormones are also nicknamed the amnestic hormones because of their capacity to wipe out existing neuronal connections and learned behavior, which in turn opens a whole new window of opportunity to learn new behavior to form new attachments. Hence the massive neuronal reorganization. You see, nature through this hormone is helping us to adapt to this huge new challenge and all the different new things we'll have to learn, from wiping butts and changing diapers to finding new resources and making new connections with all the parents and caretakers, to functioning under heavy stress due to crying and heavy sleep deprivation.

Personally, I remember vividly when my son was born. You know, for the next couple of weeks. I was on a cloud. I mean my life and all my priorities were turned upside down and I felt as if the world wasn't big enough to contain all my joy and happiness. I was boosted, turbocharged and ready to take on whatever would come my way. That I know now was a result of a massive injection of vasopressin rushing through my system.

I was on top of the world. I'm the king of the world. Woohoo! The neuroscience for parents will be about both You, the parent, and your child. Both impact each other, both influence each other and affect each other. Understanding this development, this interaction and its consequences, will help you on so many levels. What are we going to learn from this book?

Well first how to stay calm and keep control of our own emotions whenever a situation is getting out of hand. How to recognize what part of our child's brain is active and adapt our communication accordingly. How to act and react appropriately to help our child develop a strong and balanced personality. In this book we'll go from the newborn baby to the young adult.

I will give you the keys to understanding why your child is behaving in a certain way and more importantly how to react to it. I will help you grow their self-esteem, develop a stable worldview, foster their natural talents. Help them deal with bullying and peer pressure. Oh, and there are a couple of things you as a parent mt2ttt2t

should avoid at all costs and that you might not even be aware of. Keep reading, we are getting there. Let's start, sharpen your mind.

1.2 How to Learn from this Book

Now, plenty of studies have shown that couples without children are happier than couples with children. That's a bummer, right? And you just hoped that I would give you a pep talk about how great it is to be a parent. It's not going to happen. Parenting is hard. It really is. So why even bother having kids?

I mean, between the diapers, the sleepless nights, the arguments with your partner, the arguments with your kids, the stress, anxiety, that sometimes I think, if we would have known exactly how it would be like to be a parent, there would be way less children walking around. Don't pretend to be shocked by what I'm saying.

And it was so easy. Why did you buy a book on parenting in the first place, huh?

Right now, there is a silver lining here. And you might want to remember this next time your kid gets on your nerves. The good news is that all these studies on parental happiness have focused on those parents whose children still live at home. A new recent study, however, went further and also included parents whose children had already moved out. As it turns out in the long run, when their kids can take care of themselves, then their parents are happier than couples without children.

So, yes, it's all going to be worth it in the end. All the sweat and tears, it will all be worth it. It's not a promise, but a nice perspective to have. In the meantime, I'm here to help you. You might wonder why it is so hard to be a parent? Why can't we just explain to the kids how to coexist together and cooperate and live happily ever after? Why isn't that the thing?

Well, you know why. Basically, it comes down to the brains. The brain of a child is not the same as the brain of an adult. It doesn't function the same way. But different parts of the brain are active in a child which leads to different thinking processes and behaviors than in an adult. They don't follow the same reasoning. They don't make sense to us. And we, we don't make sense to them. We're basically playing the same game, but with different rules once and for all.

Kids are not adults, and we shouldn't treat them as such. Once you understand that, your life becomes a whole lot easier. Well, it doesn't, but at least things make much more sense. Of course, we will be talking about the brain and its different structures. But no worries. The main focus will always be what's in it for you. Meaning concretely, what about the brain structure is relevant for you as a parent.

This book will broadly follow the neurocognitive and behavioral approach or NBA. However, this book is not a book on the neurocognitive and behavioral approach. It's, of course, on parenting. Using the NBA as a tool. However, to do so, you will need some basics on the NBA. Having said that, I need to address one thing. I don't want to become too technical or focused too much on the geography of this or that part of the brain because there's still so much, we don't know.

Second, the different parts of the brain are highly interconnected and work together. And last but not least, in the end it doesn't really matter. We can argue for an hour that, for example, the first brain structure, the primitive brain, is responsible, as we will see in a couple of minutes, for the survival of the individual. If I want to become technical, I will have to start explaining that its mostly executing orders coming from the limbic amygdala and the hypothalamus, but it's also interconnected with the neocortex.

Very soon I will be having endless discussions about what the impact is of the dorsolateral prefrontal cortex. You will be lost. Nobody will care. And in the end, as I said, it doesn't really matter, at least here, because we don't need to go into the nuances and details. This means, I might oversimplify some things at some points, but for the sake of argument and better understanding, it's a sacrifice I'm willing to make.

My aim is for you to get more out of this book this way. I will start each section with a general lecture on brain structure. We will cover the material not from a parent's perspective, but from a general perspective. What is brain structure, what is it for, and how it operates? The chapters after that will dive into the implications of this brain structure for our children and ourselves as their parents.

So basically, with every section, I will give you the basics. You need to get you up to speed and understand the different concepts explained. So, in section two, we will cover the primitive brain, the oldest part of our brain. From an evolutionary point of view, here we will cover several of our instincts and how they play out in our kids.

In section three, we will go over the Limbic brain, still an old part of our brain in terms of evolution. Here we will see things like confidence and trust and how the interaction with others shapes our children. In Section four, we covered the Neo limbic brain. This part is very exciting as this is the brain center of our emotions and motivations which ultimately lead to our personality.

In Section five, we reached a neocortex. This is magical stuff, biological, hi tech. This is where all our executive functions are. All our more advanced thinking skills are located on all four levels. I will give you concrete advice on how to interact with your child, help him or her manage their emotions, adapt your communication to their level of understanding, and ultimately stimulate their brain so that you as a parent can really make a difference and guide your child to become the best version of itself.

Finally, in the last section, we will bring everything together and wrap things up. Sharpen your mind.

2.1 The Reptilian Brain

The first brain structure we will be looking at is the reptilian brain. It's located deep inside the skull. It's the home of our individual survival instincts and is responsible for dealing with life threatening situations, to be technically correct. It works closely together with the limbic amygdala, which is located in the next brain structure and covered in the next lecture.

The term reptilian brain refers to the erroneous belief that we inherited this part of the brain from our reptilian ancestors. Now this is incorrect. However, as amphibians and fish also shared this part of the brain, we most probably must go back to our common evolutionary ancestor of all vertebrates. The other thing with the reptilian denomination is that this part of the brain's only concern is its own individual survival.

Now, I know. I know it's unfortunate. Just to name one, some crocodiles take care of their offspring by letting them hide in their mouth for all these reasons. That's part of the brain is sometimes also referred to as the primitive brain. Anyway, just to be clear, we do not have an actual reptilian brain in our head. It's an image being used here.

The reptilian brain has three and only three ways of responding to a threat. You're probably already familiar with the famous fight or flight response. Actually, there is one more flight, fight or freeze. So back in the Stone Age, when a caveman would notice his being followed by a pack of hungry wolves, three things would happen. Now, as the first strategy our cavemen would try to outrun the wolfs, however they are pretty fast.

Our legs may be longer, but they got four of them. So, outrunning them is pretty much impossible. Second option for cavemen is to fight them off if the danger is not too strong. This could actually work sometimes. It's enough to intimidate the wolves by making ourselves look bigger, making much noise, throwing stuff around. Unfortunately, we're in the Stone Age so much more than sticks and stones won't be available. And the wolves, well, there are a lot of them. They got claws and sharp teeth and strong jaws. They are definitely not looking good.

Last but not least, our caveman can freeze. This means he makes himself as small as possible, so the threat won't see him or won't find him interesting enough as lunch. The best survival option for our caveman, though, would have been to find a big tree and climb up there hoping the wolves with get tired and eventually walk away.

So here we are 30,000 years later, and there aren't that many packs of wolves or any other hungry predators, for that matter, running around in our big cities or even in the countryside. So great. No more need for the reptilian brain. Well, not quite. In our modern lives, the reptilian brain still gets activated in situations of life or death, even if these are quite few. If you're crossing the street and a car comes right at you, you will have the same instinctive reactions as our caveman.

The first reaction is to jump away or flee. In the second phase. You might consider stopping the car with both your hands like Superman does. However, that might not work. The third reaction is to freeze like a rabbit caught in the spotlight at night. You'll just stop moving altogether. If you're lucky, the car might miss you. But our reptilian brain also gets activated when our life is not in danger. And that, ladies and gentlemen, is what today we call stress.

Stress is a defense mechanism to a perceived danger. Now, I didn't say danger, I said perceived danger because humans are probably the only species capable of worrying about something that might never happen anyway. So, when we feel stressed, we actually still use those same three strategies as our friend, the caveman. The flight becomes anxiety.

Ever felt nervous before a test or when you had to give a presentation? That is a fight stress. Fighting becomes aggressivity. Did you ever come home after a nerve-wracking day at the office, and you started shouting at the kids or your partner over something trivial? That is the fight, stress in action.

Finally, the freeze stress becomes helplessness and a face-to-face daunting task where you didn't even know where to begin. Only thinking about it made you feel depressed. Well, that is the freeze stress. So, to summarize the reptilian brain, this brain structure is responsible for our individual survival instincts, when activated, we feel stress which can take three forms flight, fight or freeze or translated in our modern world, anxiety, aggressivity or helplessness. Sharpen your mind.

2.2 The Reptilian Baby

When a child is born into this world, his brain is not, as one would like to think, a blank sheet, or no. On the contrary, a newborn has far more connections in its brain than any adult could ever have. What happens next is some kind of neural Armageddon, where during the first three months of the baby's life, around 90 percent of the neural connections of the limbic territories just disappear in a selective way based on the interactions with the surroundings.

It's as if our brain was wired to be able to adapt to any possible situations. And once it's establishing what will be useful, it just gets rid of the excess baggage. With a newborn, the brain isn't fully operational yet, some parts are just plainly immature. There is one part, though, that is fully operational and that is the reptilian brain. As we saw before, the reptilian brain switches on when we are facing a perceived danger for the newborn baby.

Everything is a potential threat, and the slightest discomfort will trigger the reptilian brain. Hungry danger, too much light danger, too cold danger. Mommy's not around danger. I don't know 'where am I' - danger. There's a stranger in the room - danger. I just peed myself. Danger. I could go on like that on and on, but you get the picture. The baby responds each time. By crying. Now, you must understand one important thing about babies. The only way they must communicate is by crying.

So don't interpret every time they cry as being sad. No, they're not. Remember, there are three reptilian strategies. Flight, fight and freeze. Sometimes their cries will mean different things. Get me out of this or flee response. I'm angry because I'm hungry or a fight response. Or I'm scared. Where's my mommy? Or a freeze response.

So that's a tricky thing with babies. When we hear someone cry or the first reaction is to offer comfort and free them from stress, not flee or fight. It's no use to comfort a wet baby. That baby needs to get a clean diaper, not a lullaby. Did you ever try to comfort a baby just to see him turn even more red and cry even harder. Congratulations. That was a fine stress response which includes babies who want to win their fight.

You want the baby to calm down, give him what he or she wants. OK, I must add here that this is only valid for small babies. Once the baby reaches the socializing age, it's important not to give in to everything they want but will dive into that in the next chapter about to paleo limbic brain. For now, remember that before two years of age, when in fact stress, the best way to calm them is to give them what they want.

As we will see later, this reptilian brain plays a very important role in defining who we will become in terms of personality and motivation. It's the ground floor of all our emotions and will continue to play an important role during all our life. All our survival instincts are here, and even when we are not in situations of life or death, feeling stress will be the best indicator that our reptilian brain is active. Yes, stress. When our reptilian brain is active, we feel stress.

So, can babies feel stress? Yes. The children experience stress. What about young adults? Absolutely, yes. It's not about the amount of pressure we feel or worries we have or work that we must do. Stress is a physical reaction to a perceived danger. That perceived danger can be pressure, worries or work, but it can be the most trivial of things like a broken doll or children playing rough, never judge the emotional pain of someone else.

What we believe to be a catastrophe is, in our experience, a catastrophe, especially with kids. Why? Well, it has everything to do with our ability to put things into perspective. That ability is a realm of our prefrontal brain, which is the last one to mature from roughly seventeen years old onward. It is sufficiently developed to avoid being traumatized by humiliation and related experiences. But it will only reach full maturity until we reach 24 years of age. Yes. Twenty-four.

From the brain's perspective, we become adults at 24 years old. This is because of this late maturity of the brain that children are so vulnerable on an emotional level, they can get really hurt and even traumatized for life. And they don't have the tools yet of the prefrontal brain to deal with strong, overwhelming emotions.

How to recognize the reptilian brain is active. Flight, fight and freeze. Flight is all about movement and avoiding confrontation. When you're moralizing your kid and see how he's avoiding your eyes and constant negation. That's a pure flee reaction.

Fighting is about overpowering and winning. Tension builds up and shows, especially in the jaws. The arms and the legs have seen your kids stamping its feet. Or do you recognize this fight?

For kids, stress freeze is all about looking for protection. It's usually tears. However, another strong indicator is the lack of desire, total apathy. If your child doesn't want to do anything anymore, their mind shuts down. Something fishy is going on.

So how do we deal with the stress of children? Well, if you follow official NBA guidelines, you should always show the person in front of you that you are on their side. You go with the flow. That means something different for all three strategies with fleeing, you give options, you crack a joke, make them laugh. With fighting, you don't fight back. You share their outrage saying things like, if I were you, I would be furious. Now, if the kid is angry because of something you did at least acknowledge their feelings, say things like, I understand you're angry right now or you have the right to be angry.

With freezing, you give support. No pep talks needed. Just being there is often enough. That leads me to my favorite stress relief strategy. It works well, especially with smaller children, as one can quickly jump from one stress response to another. It's sometimes difficult and confusing to pick the right answer, especially when my own kids are angry or frustrated. I could feel intuitively that just acknowledging their emotions was not enough.

So, I did an experiment that worked like magic. I started what I call my own a hug response. Whenever one of my kids shows signs of stress, regardless of if it's flight, fight or freeze, I offer them a hug. Now, a hug would typically work with freezing and not with fleeing or fighting. I still offered to hug and if they say no, I tell them that if they want one later, it will still be available.

At first, I must admit it was difficult for me to offer a hug when one of my kids was fighting me. When someone fights you. Your instinct is to fight back, not start cuddling. My children as well were surprised that a hug was an option at that point. Eventually they would come to me and accept the hug. Now, over time I saw how the time between fighting and hug shrank up to the time that now we hardly fight anymore. And they come asking for a hug before we even fight has been a great way to deal with life's little everyday frustrations that may occasionally arise.

The reason why hugging is so effective is that it releases oxytocin in our body, oxytocin is sometimes called the bonding hormone. It facilitates the development of trust and attachment between individuals, exactly the kind of relationship you want with your child. So even if you're not the hugging type, I strongly recommend hugging your kids as often as you can, even when you fight. Sorry, let me rephrase that. Especially when you have a fight. Oxytocin slows down the heart rate and decreases blood pressure, which is exactly what both of you need in such a situation.

So now I can hear you think, come on, you can't be serious when you say that you have to hug your kids and give them what they want whenever they get angry. Well, that is not what I said. This you should do, when the reptilian brain is active. Remember that the reptilian brain switches on when faced with a perceived danger. In other words, it's a defense mechanism. Fighting stress is defensive aggression. However, when the Paralimbic is switched on, as we will see in the next lecture, it's a different game altogether. Sharpen your mind.

2.3 On Movement

So far, we've seen that this primitive brain oversees our survival instincts, right? We can safely fight or freeze. So that's it? No, not quite. There's so much more to this region of the brain. It's named a primitive brain or reptilian brain indicates a lack of sophistication. But that's not the case. You know, the name refers to an evolutionary perspective. It's the oldest part of the brain. From an evolutionary point of view, this doesn't mean that its function is primitive. A better name would have been the primal brain as an essential or fundamentally essential.

Yes, because it regulates our heart rate, our breathing, our body temperature, even our movements, sleep and more. Without it, we would simply not be able to live. Which brings us to one of my favorite theories about the brain, and it answers the very simple and crucial question why do we even have a brain in the first place?

Now, think about that for a second. Why do we have a brain? Well, what if I told you, it is not for thinking, knowing all these existential questions about the meaning of life? Who am I? Why am I here, to be or not to be? That's just a side product of collateral, if you want, derived from the core function. The very reason why we have a brain is to move. I'm in shock right now, the main purpose is movement.

And when you think of it, it makes so much sense because plants, trees and flowers don't have a brain and don't move, and some animals, even those who only wiggle, have developed the beginning of a nervous system to coordinate all that wiggling. Now look at our brain. And what do we see as a part of this primitive brain? I mean, in the primal brain in the back of our skull will find the cerebellum. Cerebellum means small brain, and it's located right on top of our spinal cord. It evolved some 400 million years ago. Just to put that into perspective, modern human beings, Homo sapiens has been on Earth for only about three hundred thousand years.

So, 400 million years is really old. This cerebellum represents only 10 percent of our brain's volume that holds about 50 percent of the neurons in our entire brain, 50 percent. And you'll never guess what the cerebellum means. It's called a little brain. Exactly. We're talking balance, muscle coordination of movement and motor learning. And in newborn babies, not surprisingly, it is a part of the brain that will grow most in the first three months while they wiggle and move and learn the very basics of how this whole movement thing works.

So, movement is the very reason why we have a brain in the first place. What do we do with our kids? Hmm? We send them to school, teach them to sit down the whole day when they come back from school. We put them in front of the TV because, let's face it, is the best and cheapest babysitter around. We criticize our children because they don't sit still.

Newsflash, kids aren't made to sit still. It is our modern lifestyle in our society's expectations towards kids that are the problem, not our kids not being able to sit still. That's normal. That's healthy. That's how it's supposed to be. If the very reason why we evolved the brain in the first place is to coordinate movement, it is movement and a lot of it which is key to developing a strong and healthy brain in those young kids.

Let them move, let them play, let them get dirty, for crying out loud. Kick them out of your house. Let them run in the garden, send them to a sports club. Literally anything is better than having them sit in front of the tv for hours. I'll talk about screens later, by the way, but this one is not negotiable. Movement is key. Movement is the first pillar to develop a healthy brain in your child's. Sharpen your mind.

2.4 On climbing trees

Quick side note on climbing trees, so I know I just gave that example about how you should let your kids try things out and don't let your fears withhold them from doing things like, for example, climbing trees. Now, about that specifically that it turns out that climbing trees is ridiculously good for our brain. Yeah, I know. Who would have thought, right. A recent study showed an amazing 50 percent boost in working memory.

You know, the thing is like climbing up a tree with each step there is a boost. Our brain has to continuously update its model of the immediate surroundings, making our brain work much harder. It's not only climbing trees actually. It works also for other dynamic activities, like balancing on a beam, carrying awkward weights and navigating around obstacles.

By involving ourselves in activities that are unpredictable and require us to consciously adapt our movements, we can boost our working memory to perform better, which means the next time your kids want to climb a tree, not only shouldn't you stop them, but you should seriously consider joining them.

2.5 On Food

Our primitive, primal brain is also in charge of food, or indirectly at least, since digestion happens in our stomach and intestines. But it's the hypothalamus via various mechanisms which control appetite and food intake. It is also responsible for the control of hunger and thirst. Yes, appetite from your newborn baby crying to get its next meal to your adolescent insatiable appetite. It all comes from this little bugger.

The sense of taste gets processed in the neocortex. But the sense of hunger is its motivation. You see, it's all about survival at this level of the brain. The feeling of hunger and thirst is the unpleasant reminder to make sure we eat and drink enough, as without it we end up dying. And from a great perspective, it's even more true. Our primal brain represents only two percent of our whole brain. Its weight produces 20 percent of its energy.

So, food intake, also known as energy source, is vital for our brain to function well. And water or liquid at least? Well, our brain consists of 73 percent water, so I rest my case, but it's about more than that. You see, food provides us with the very building blocks for our brain. When we take out the water, our brain consists of fat, and the highest quality of fat around is Omega 3. You know, to one we've been bombarded with Omega three marketing. Well, it turns out Omega 3 is not only a marketing trick to have us buy more of a certain product.

Omega 3 is essential to our diets as our body does not produce it. So, we need to get it out of our food. Where do we get Omega 3? Well, you know, from fish, yes, but not any fish, fatty fish such as salmon, herring, sardines, etc. nuts are considered the best. I love these nuts because when you open them, they look like a brain. I'm sorry. That's just me, gee king out here. OK, what else? Milk and eggs. Yes, but not all milk and eggs. This is interesting.

If the animal, the cow or chicken got its food from freely grazing around, then the milk or eggs will contain Omega 3. But if, on the contrary, they were fed mass industrial food, you know, they wouldn't produce Omega 3. Basically, we try to "improve" nature and it gives us the middle finger. I love that. Now there is more. Of course. I put a list with Omega 3 rich food at the end of the book. I'm not sure you realize that not all fats are good for the brain, right? Fast food, pizza and burgers where you see the grease dripping off. Yeah. Knowing that's not going to be good for us is important.

We have to go for a balanced diet, ideally Mediterranean style food, with olive oil and lots of fresh fruit and vegetables. Healthy food is another one of the pillars for a healthy brain. Now, we as parents, we educate our kids. Much of the food we eat is acquired taste, meaning we get used to it and that's why we like it. If you never serve broccoli to your kids, they won't like it. If you serve it weekly, they will eventually make sure they have a predisposition to prefer something which tastes sweet.

However, that doesn't stop them from being able to like real food as well. Here we need to be role models. If we want our kids to eat healthy, we have to eat healthy and serve them proper food. OK, that's all great and dandy, but that's for the kids and adolescents, right? What about babies who don't want to eat salmon or nuts, let alone broccoli? Well, I thought you'd never ask. OK, so the important thing to understand here is that from conception onward, our brain is creating neurons and brain cells at a dizzying rate.

Our kids are literally building their brain. It gradually slows down. But the beginnings of truly impressive the brain grows at a rate of about 250,000 nerve cells per minute on average throughout pregnancy. In the first 90 days, only three months, newborn babies brain goes from thirty three percent to fifty five percent of an adult's brain size. That is huge. The amount of new brain cells that need to be produced is just gigantic.

The building blocks for this huge undertaking is the Omega 3. Well, where does it come from exactly? Mother milk. Now, just to show you the importance of this, a 2014 study has shown a clear link between mother milk and academic success. Their findings show that the amount of Omega 3 acids in a mother's milk is the strongest predictor of test performance, and it outweighs national income and the number of dollars spent per pupil in schools.

Now, where does the mother get Omega 3 from? Remember, we don't produce it ourselves, right? So that leaves us with only one source of Omega 3, the mother's diet. Depending on what the mother eats, the baby will get Omega 3 through breastfeeding. Now, those first weeks and months are crucial for brain development. Before you start giving tons of pills to your kids, you must know that supplements don't seem to work. And the best intake is still from natural sources like fatty fish, etc.

Now, I'm telling you all this regarding the positive impact of Omega 3, but the opposite is true as well. You can really harm your baby's brain in its development through, for example, the intake of alcohol. Ever wondered why you shouldn't drink alcohol when you're pregnant?

Well, I can't speak for other organs, but regarding the brain, alcohol is a no go.

You must understand that alcohol dramatically slows down neurogenesis. So, what are the effects of alcohol on a fetus or a newborn? Well, in those early days when the brain undergoes a stellar growth rate, and you basically pull the brakes. Yeah, no, no, that's not good. It's a one-way ticket to cognitive impairment or worse. Now, I know some of us have conceived in a state of slight inebriation, also known as totally harmless. I've had worried mums confessing to me all kinds of sins.

There's too much information regarding that, but don't worry. At conception, we're talking one cell splitting in two cells and four cells, then eight cells. Well, you know the story. You know how it goes at this point. There was no differentiation yet of the cells. There are no brain cells yet, so no active neurogenesis to be tampered with. Oh, and while we're on the topic of diet and drinks, get rid of sugar.

My kids don't drink sodas, at least not when I'm around. We never go to fast foods. In the last 10 years, we went only once. Actually, we were abroad in the middle of nowhere and it was lunchtime and there were no other restaurants anywhere near anyway. Why am I so drastic on sugar? Well, for starters, sugar slows down neurogenesis, the creation of new neurons. You don't want that.

Second, sugar has drug like effects in the reward center of the brain, the famous dopamine. On top of that, excessive sugar consumption leads to memory and cognitive deficiencies. Last but not least, research shows that eating high sugar diets impairs impulsive control. That's your kid not being able to control him or herself. And I'm not even talking about weight gain, obesity, diabetes or dental decay.

Here, a balanced diet rich in Omega 3, eliminating sugar and saturated fats is one more of those fundamental pillars for a healthy brain. Mental note to self. Sharpen your mind.

2.6 Sleep

In the last lecture, I was talking about how the hypothalamus regulates appetite. In this one, I want to focus on another function vital to this small but powerful brain structure. And this one is probably, if I had to choose the most important cornerstone for a healthy brain, is sleep. Now, there are many things we can do as parents to help and guide our children. And by far without any competition coming close, the number one is sleep.

Yes, you heard that right. Make sure your child sleeps enough. This is true for absolutely everybody. So that includes you as a parent, but even more so for our children. Let me explain. We adults sleep on average eight hours a night, children even more so. Now think about it. We're extremely vulnerable when we sleep. We're at the mercy of predators and yet we all sleep for about one third of our life. That is huge. It's more than any other activity we do.

So, it must be pretty important from an evolutionary perspective. Sleep must give us an advantage so big that after all these years, we're still using it every day. That evolution decided to keep this feature. But sleep has a bad press. It is often seen as a waste of time, especially in our modern lives, where we're all so busy and we regularly walk around sleep deprived. Many people boast about how little they sleep. It's not good. There are many reasons why we sleep. Funny enough, physical rest isn't that important on that list.

Our body and muscles could do with only a couple of hours of rest in one day. The main reason for sleep is in our brain and has nothing to do with rest. At some points in our sleep, our brain is more active than when we were awake. You see, at night a rerun takes place of all types of maintenance tasks and upgrades to our brain. We're talking about organizing information, removal of toxins and also especially for younger individuals, construction and maturation processes.

That's why the younger the child, the more it sleeps, that's why a baby spends around 14 hours a day sleeping, it's literally constructing its brain and will continue to do so for years to come. At five years old, we're talking 11 hours of sleep. Nine years old should not have less than 10 hours of sleep at night. The brain of adolescents goes through a serious maturation process which starts at the back of the brain and ends up with the prefrontal lobes in the front.

This process, also called myelination, takes years to accomplish and is extremely important. Basically, it's a fundamental upgrade of all wiring, making the existing connections faster and better insulated. And that's why our adolescents spend so much time in their bed. No, they're not lazy. Their brain is doing some serious remodeling up there and it's working overtime. If your teenager isn't sleeping at least eight to 10 hours a night, he or she will be underperforming.

There have been studies, many studies, about the effect of sleep deprivation on the brain. And the results are pretty dramatic. You know, just remember how you were as a parent when you first had your baby. Remember how you ended up sleep deprived, and you just couldn't function normally anymore? Well, the same happens to our children when they don't sleep enough. By now, there is a mountain of studies showing a direct link between sleep and academic performance.

Long story short, well, if our kids don't sleep enough, it will be hard for them to focus. If they don't focus, they won't be able to hear or remember what has been said. But it goes further, you know, with lack of sleep. It's the memory consolidation process that gets affected and thus with a weaker memory, their academic performance gets affected. You know, this is just focusing on memory because our brain regulates pretty much everything we do. And poor sleep impacts all aspects of our well-being and affects our health, both short term and long term.

And it's not only our physical health. Poor sleep is linked to anxiety and depression, but also aggression. Studies have shown how a lack of sleep impacts our amygdala, making it bigger and more sensitive. Now you must know that the amygdala is our brain center of fear and aggression. So, that's why when we don't sleep enough, we become easily irritated, annoyed, stressed and aggressive. If your kid is throwing tantrums, being moody or even aggressive, this is the first place to check. Is he or she sleeping enough?

Now, I do realize that as much as we would like them to go to sleep, it's easier said than done. Right? Lucky for us, there are several things we can do to help our children sleep. And at different ages, different strategies apply with babies. Well, falling asleep is all about a ritual. A warm bath before going to bed is soothing and helps a lot with toddlers. Reading a bedtime story or singing a nursery rhyme works magic as well. It is very important to create a fixed ritual so the child knows it's almost time to go to sleep and their brain will start to prepare for the night to come.

Putting your kid to sleep every night around the same time is also very helpful, as they will develop a predictable schedule and a sleep routine which will help them for years to come. Because once they reach adolescence, it is the sleep discipline which will make a difference. I said before, an ever-growing number of studies show how there is a direct link between sleep and academic performance. If your teenager doesn't do well at school, the very first place to look at his sleep patterns. It is his or her lack of sleep.

Many youngsters don't sleep enough during the week and end up oversleeping on the weekend as to catch up on the lack of sleep, they'd build up during the week. Right now, while this may seem like a good idea at first, it's making things worse. You see, it's not only the amount of sleep that impacts the grades, but also the regularity behind it. It's going to sleep and wake up at approximately the same time. It's as important as the number of hours one sleeps.

There's an interesting explanation for this. You see, it is very possible that it's not the regularity itself which makes a difference, but the underlying self-discipline it takes to go to bed, which is also impacting academic performance. It is this self-discipline which makes the youngster good at school and ends up going to bed at a regular time. Now, the interesting part is, if your son or daughter doesn't show self-discipline, a good way to start developing it is by going to bed every night, that's more or less the same time and thus creating that healthy sleeping pattern. Any way you look at it, you score. Sharpen your mind.

2.7 On Co-sleeping

I must admit, at times, it's anything but comfortable once I woke up with my son's foot on my face. Oh, don't ask. Yes, you will wake up 20 times and yes, you will be tired the next morning. Yes, you will most probably get hit by them as they turn around in their sleep. So, sleeping with your kids is mostly not about having a good night's sleep, at least for the parents.

So, we have established that it's bad for you. How is that for them? I've heard of people claiming that it would develop an unhealthy bond between parents and child. What? Come on. Look, let me put it in a very simple way. We human beings are the only mammals who are not sleeping with our children. All the others do, without exception. Some critics now believe children grow up to be insecure and more reliant on their parents.

Well studies show exactly the opposite. In fact, babies and toddlers who are less likely to have behavioral problems, are because children have strong ties with their parents as they venture out into unknown. If anything happens, they know they can rely on their parents. That gives them the confidence to do things, to try new things. Their parents are their safe haven where they can return to at any time. That's what makes a child's spirit strong.

And sleeping together can be part of that. Now, don't get me wrong, I'm not saying that you must sleep with your kids. I'm just telling you that it's more than OK to do so. It's equally

OK not to do so if your child doesn't feel the need for it. There's one important note, though, watch out for small babies. A recent British study showed that babies who sleep with their parents have five times higher risk of sudden infant death syndrome. Keep the baby close to you next to your bed, but don't share the bed with them.

Now, of course, the other mammals don't have to go to work the next morning as we do, so it would be wise to find a way to combine both. My wife and I have installed a very simple rule that is clear to everyone, and maybe it can help you as well. Rule states that everyone falls asleep in his or her own bed. If one wakes early, even if that's the middle of the night, you can come to mommy and daddy. But we fall asleep in our own bed.

Of course, sometimes the little one still insists on falling asleep in our bed, but we stay firm and calm to rule is simple to understand. So, it doesn't last long before they give in. Because if you establish a rule, don't make exceptions afterwards. It's hell to get them to comply. So don't feel guilty. There's absolutely no reason whatsoever for that. Sharpen your mind.

3.1 The Paleo limbic Brain

The second brain structure of interest to us is the Paleo limbic brain. This is the home of some of our unconscious scripts inherited from our education, which regulate our life. Where two reptilian brains were aimed at the survival of the individual, the Paleo limbic brain is responsible for the survival of the group. Now, scientists used to believe that in evolutionary terms, it developed with the emergence of the first mammals who decided to live in huts. That is not correct, however, as it is also found with other vertebrates besides the question of its origins.

Its purpose is clear - living together maximizes chances of survival of a group. However, social life needed to be regulated in order to do so. The Paleo limbic brain defines the position of the individual towards the group. This translates into two key concepts that are regulated here. Our self-confidence and our trust in others. So, self-confidence and trust, we put them on a two-sided axis. In the middle, we will find assertiveness here. An individual finds balance. He or she doesn't have too much self-confidence or trust. Neither does he or she like it.

Now, wait a minute. Too much self-confidence? How can someone have so much confidence? Well, it's all a matter of words or semantics, if you will. With the neurocognitive and behavioral approach, we defined a tipping point where confidence in oneself turns into overconfidence. I am entitled to more than others. This belief that we are better for whatever reason may be because we have more money, better looks, a bigger car, whatever that belief is for us. Too much self-confidence. Once we agree on the words that we speak about same concepts, we can work with them. So, in the middle, we have assertiveness.

Here, people can say yes to things they want and refuse, things they don't want. Too much self-confidence is what we call dominance now. Dominance is not, as one may think about yelling and overpowering the other, but it is its mild form. It's all about manipulation and seduction. The dominant person can be very charming and nice. The thing is, it's not genuine. They do so to obtain favors to get what they want for the dominant person. Others are evaluated in terms of utility. They will use them to obtain their goal, whatever that may be, in its most extreme form. Excessive self-confidence leads to a narcissistic personality disorder.

A lack of self-confidence we call submissiveness. Submissiveness is a real burden. Whenever something turns out well, they feel they were lucky. If something goes wrong, the submissive person will feel it's their fault. If you compare that to a dominant person, every success they feel is their doing and failure is always due to others. The dominant person is totally incapable of admitting mistakes or taking responsibility, as in their opinion, they are so superior to everyone else.

In its most extreme form, submissiveness will lead to melancholic depression. On the opposite side to one of trust in others, we will call someone who is lacking trust all together to the point of being marginal. You've probably heard about conspiracy theories. Did you know that four percent of the population of the United States actually believes that shapeshifting reptilian people control our world by taking on the human form and control our governments? This is a good example of what marginality looks like in its extreme form. It turns into paranoia.

Too much trust in others we will call X-Reality. Have you ever received mail from people claiming to need your help to free large sums of money of which you would receive your share? Of course. Now, over the years, this one has known many versions from a bank to the lottery and even political dissidents. I once received a mail, supposedly from the daughter of Colonel Gadhafi, the dictator of Libya. These, of course, are scams.

An assertive person wonders Who would ever fall for that. Well, actually many people do. They have excessive trust in others, which leads to gullibility? The people sending out those emails know that their mail isn't intended for assertive people. They prey on those among us who trust in its most extreme form. Actuality becomes mystical delirium.

The Paleo limbic is quite an archaic structure of the brain. It can learn and evolve. However, it does so very slowly. Any person with a lack of self-confidence could testify. It's not something you can solve. Over the weekend, any person claiming to be able to grow your self-esteem in a record time is a fraud. It is a physical impossibility. The Paleo limbic brain cannot evolve that fast. It has never been observed until now. The only exception to this rule is traumatizing events, which can shatter your self-confidence in seconds. However, a quick shift is always downwards, never upwards.

We can recognize when the Paleo limbic brain is active when the reptilian brain is operative because people react and treat stress differently. We will see people behaving in a very territorial way. It's all about power games. Above all, it's a dominant behavior that is the most problematic. It's actually quite easy to spot.

It goes from peacock or macho behavior over bullying to all types of harassment. I said before these people never question their own behavior and never learn.

There is good news, though. Just as in the animal kingdom, it is rare to find alpha males fighting to death over a female or a hood. They will try to impress and intimidate. Sometimes they will actually fight. However, fights usually don't last long. It's more probing and trying, checking out the strength of the other. Once it's established, the other one is stronger, they will disengage.

Why? Well, getting wounded is very dangerous. Even a small wound can get infected. Predators and prey alike need to be able to run as fast as they can, so they need to minimize dangerous situations. The Paleo limbic brain works with the same logic. It tries to impress and intimidate. However, it is actually quite a coward. From the moment it feels firm resistance, it will try once, twice, maybe three times. Then it will disengage.

This is great news for people having to deal with a dominant person in their surroundings, particularly when dominance is combined with marginality. Why, you ask? Well, this combination leads easily to jealousy, which can potentially ruin a happy relationship. So, to summarize the Paleo limbic brain, this brain structure is responsible for the survival of the group and works around to access self-confidence and trust. When activated, the Paleo limbic makes us quite territorial, which can become dominant, submissive, marginal or actual. Sharpen your mind.

3.2 The Parental Instinct

Some time ago I was picking up my kids from school. Whilst crossing the street a car arrived and gently pulled the brakes letting us pass. We started crossing the street and at the same moment another car came from the same direction at full speed over taking the first one and if it wouldn't have been for my reflex to pull back my kids, they would have ended in a hospital at best or in a graveyard. Now if you knew me personally you wouldn't know I'm a very calm person who hates all types of conflicts and arguments and never uses swear words.

But oh my God... the words that came out of my mouth shouted, yelled at that driver in the middle of the street using combinations of blasphemy, anatomy and cooking modes that rarely combine in one sentence. Some other parents around covered their kids' ears and my reputation of a gentle caring dad turned into 'Don't be fooled. You don't want to mess with that guy.' Once I calmed down like three days later, I started thinking about what happened there.

This wasn't a classic fight reflex when our life is in danger because my life hadn't been in danger. My children's life had been. At the same time, it was clearly the limbic amygdala who had taken over and then it struck me. So, that's what they called a maternal/paternal instinct. You know evolution is amazing. Our children are born completely immature. A human baby cannot survive without outside help. From a brain perspective seventy percent of its growth happens after birth. Those babies and small children just don't stand a chance.

So, evolution has put a switch in our brain that only switches on when we have children or at least take care of them, and that switch is in the limbic amygdala. It is the part of the brain which triggers stress and is responsible for territorial power games. In other words, 'Those kids are mine and don't you even think about messing with them.' It pushes us to go berserk and even face head on much larger and stronger opponents, in order to keep those little ones safe.

You can witness that in numerous wildlife documentaries where desperate mothers protect their young ones from predators approaching their offspring by fearlessly attacking them. Now recent research has shown that with us humans both male and female have that switch. At least I know that I do. Now. The thing is, when the limbic amygdala is active, there's no use for rational talk. It's better to let the other person calm down first because in that mental mode you're just wasting your time trying to talk reason into the other person.

So, what about you. Have you ever felt that parental instinct to protect your kids against a potential danger?

3.3 The Paleo Limbic Toddler

That cute little reptilian baby, so helpless and fragile, does grow at an unbelievable rate, its development is beyond anything it will experience in its later life, from physical growth, maturity and coordination to emotional and cognitive development. At around two, two and a half years old, this baby enters a new, important phase of its development. Its limbic brain just got activated, and your troubles as a parent are about to begin. Ever heard about a terrible two and three of age nature?

Sometimes it's also referred to as the first adolescence. At two, two and a half years old, your toddler enters the socialization phase, he or she will start to interact with other children. Until now, whenever you would have put two babies next to each other, they would have played each on their own. Now, they start to play together, and those changes everything. Because playing together leads to sharing toys and who gets what and before you know they are biting each other or throwing things at each other's heads.

You see, the limbic brain is responsible for how we position ourselves towards others. When the limbic first switches on, the struggle for power starts, and your sweet little baby quickly turns into an adorable monster. That's what I call the gremlin stage one moment they are adorable, sweet little things, and then suddenly they turn into these evil gremlins. For your reference, whenever they turn into a gremlin, that's the power of limbic that just switched on.

Basically, your child will test you and others to see how far they can go. Now, remember how I told you to hug it out with the reptilian behavior here? No such thing. No more, Mr. Nice Guy. It is imperative that you show who's in charge. You have to stay firm in consequence. Don't start an argument. You don't start to explain things or appeal to the kids' rational capacities. A kid is not a mini adult. Your child's brain isn't mature enough to understand anyway, so don't even start explaining anything. You are in charge. No, means NO.

Why not? Because I told you so. They will start to manipulate you, tire you out too. They'll even try blackmail and intimidation. My son one day looked at his mom in the eyes and without blinking, just said, Mummy, I don't love you anymore. And then he repeated it like three times just to make sure she got the message. While dad was so harsh, I don't even remember why, but I believe it had to do with him not wanting to take his bath or something like that.

That really hurt my wife's feelings. It took a long discussion and some tears to get over it. But even then, you can't give in.

It's a power game, and it's one you don't want to lose because before you know it, they run the show. However, having said that, you should pick your battles and let your kid win from time to time. Not with important stuff, of course, but for the little things. With my daughter every morning there was a fight to get her dressed in time as she didn't want me to dress her. She wanted to do it all by herself every morning. Same battle against time that I knew we would eventually lose. Each time I would put her clothes on, she would do them off to put them back on painstakingly slowly.

Oh wow. I tried everything. I bribed her, punished her, threatened her, begged her nothing. So, I decided to accept it. Started to wake her up earlier. When she took too much time, I explained to her that we wouldn't have time anymore for breakfast. A couple of times she didn't miss breakfast, so she started to learn about the consequences of her actions. She did win that battle as she continued to get dressed at her own rhythm. And I, well, I learned to adapt to it, and it's important for self-esteem that they win some of these battles. It helps them in establishing self-worth, their assertiveness, as we will see in the next lecture.

3.4 The key to Self Confidence

As explained before, with the Paleo brain, we position ourselves towards the people around us, we're not born with this position. It's something we acquire once the paleo limbic brain switches on. When we are around two, two and a half years old for the next ten years, we start identifying and acquiring our sense of self-worth and trust towards others. After those ten years, our level of self-confidence is fixed. It can still evolve slowly. Over time, however, don't expect major shifts.

The critical year for defining our self-confidence is between two and 12 years old.

After that, you will still see a limbic outburst during adolescence, as we will see later in this book. However, the Paleo limbic positioning after puberty is very close to the one before puberty. This rebellious stage does not affect the essence of where we see ourselves in terms of our relationship with others. Needless to say, those 10 years from two to twelve are extremely important and can potentially give your child a strong handicap for the rest of their life.

I know this sounds traumatic and I apologize, as I don't want to scare you. However, do not underestimate the importance of this stage. Discipline is the key word in shaping the Paleo limbic. This brain structure has something very primal about it, almost animalistic, and it has to be tamed. However, don't overdo it as excess in both directions is harmful. When a child is raised in an environment without discipline, without limits nor rules and gets away with everything, this is what's happening.

The brain, the Paleo limbic brain learns that, hey, I can do whatever I want. Not only that, but it starts seeing all this as an instrument to obtain the things they want. Others are there to submit to do as I want and as I need. They are there for my pleasure. Before long, your kid becomes this despicable person, a little tyrant, and will remain so for the rest of its life. This leads to typical dominant behavior such as bullying, harassment, peacock or macho behavior, etc., but also manipulative behavior and a total lack of authenticity. These kinds of people typically end up alone and bitter as they are incapable of building authentic, fulfilling relationships.

Now, on the contrary, if you raise your child with too much discipline, that has consequences, too, and you constantly limit your child and don't let him do things or try out new stuff, their brain will learn that "I cannot do things alone by myself". I'm not worthy of the trust of others. I need supervision from others to do things before long. Your child ends up as this submissive, dependent, fearful little creature that will always be looking for someone else's approval.

Submissiveness is a real burden. As proof of that or the numerous books and courses to gain more self-confidence. There's a whole industry around it. Sadly, for submissive people, as the limbic brain can only evolve very slowly, there are no miracle solutions, and it would take years of positive reinforcement to overcome their lack of self-confidence.

So, what can we do as parents to discipline as bad, not enough is bad. What's left? Well, you will have to find the right balance. The trick is to define a framework within which your child can do an experiment as it pleases. However, the rules that were set up are to be non-negotiable. Any trespassing has to have consequences. You know what they say. Don't point a gun if you're not ready to shoot. Do not threaten your child with a punishment only to let him get away.

Because for your brain, when you do something, you know you shouldn't, the absence of a punishment equals a reward. In other words, you're rewarding your child for not complying and assigning him to do more of the same. At that point, you can just kiss your authority goodbye and expect an exhausting daily battle to have your children obey you.

Now, once your child reaches twelve and if the rules in your house are not clearly defined and enforced, your little gremlin will remain in its monster stage. Nonetheless, your child's limbic brain will continue to test the limits. He can act as a bully one day without that meaning he has developed into this dominant, horrible person. No, he's just testing, experimenting. His position on the axis of self-confidence will continue to fluctuate until the age of 12, after which it will remain stable.

And don't worry, it's not because you've been strict that your kid will become submissive. It's true constant reinforcement over this period of ten years that slowly but surely your child's position on the axis of self-confidence will define itself. So, relax, don't worry. You have plenty of opportunities to help your child develop a healthy dose of self-confidence. Not too much. Not too little. Just be aware of how this game is played by consequence, and everything will be fine.

3.5 Beat the Bully

When my son was only three years old, he didn't want to go to school anymore. One morning I found him in a corner of his room trying to hide from me. His whole-body language was screaming, I'm afraid. I sat down next to him and tried to find out what had happened. Eventually, I could figure out there was this kid at school who was hitting him. So, my fatherly blood boiled. I could already see me lecturing his father about bad parenting and so on.

So, one hour later, I was talking with my son's kindergarten teacher. She acknowledged the bullying. It wasn't only my son who was a victim, but it seemed to be quite random and widespread to my horror. She added that for sure, my kid would often be picked upon as he has a very gentle nature, is quite introverted and shy, in other words, an ideal target to be ravaged. All these images came to me where you see that one kid who gets bullied around is capable of standing up for himself.

Well, that kid apparently was my son. I came home in despair. I talked to my wife about it. So, what could we do? They would most probably be in the same class for the next nine years or so. The perfect scenario to turn my boy into a submissive person. So, what were the options? She wanted to send him to some kind of martial arts lessons. I wanted to teach him how to run faster. We even thought about changing school.

Then I turned to the neurocognitive and behavioral approach. I was supposed to be this behavioral expert, knowing how the brain works and how it impacts our behavior. And then this happened to my own son for sure. There had to be a way that I could help him. I'm a pacifist. So, teaching him to hit back was not an option, especially because otherwise his little sister could end up paying the bill. Telling him to go to the teacher each time the bully would bother him wasn't good enough either, as that would take power away from him.

I had to find a way where he could be in charge of his own destiny. So, I dove deep into neurocognitive and behavioral approach. I looked for ways to translate all this neuroscientific stuff into a simple language and method that my son could understand and apply. Bullying is dominant limbic behavior. It's all about intimidation. If intimidation doesn't work, it stops. So. Suddenly I had an idea.

I called my son and told him we would play a game; we did like half an hour of intensive role play where I taught him to stand as tall as possible, look angry and say, no, no, no. While pointing a finger to me, I explained to him he had to do that to his bully. The next time he would bother him, after that half hour where we laughed a lot, and I saw him grow in confidence. I will let it rest for the next couple of weeks. I didn't hear anything about the bully anymore.

It wasn't until two weeks later that I found him hiding again, the bully again. I asked him if he had done the no, no, no thing, and he said he didn't. So, we did another session of roleplay. The week after that, his teacher called me when I picked him up from school. She said she wanted to tell me something that had happened that day. She told me how she saw how the bully took a toy away from my son and that he, my son stood up, pointed his finger at him and started saying with a loud voice, no, no, no. The bully just gave the toy back, turned around and left him.

She said she was so proud of him, that she had no idea how I felt at that moment. Since that day, there has been no bullying anymore. But still, my wife and I decided to take this one step further. My wife had this brilliant idea to invite a bully to our house. At first, I looked at her with unbelief. I said, like, you want to invite that kid, he is like the devil incarnate. I mean, he's the enemy. He's not entering our home. Think about it. She said, we invite him over, they play together, they become buddies. He stops bullying him.

I was speechless. I mean, this was Machiavellian and brilliant. Totally twisted, though, but full of sense. At the same time, I was in awe, and it worked. It worked like a charm. Not only did the bullying stop completely, but they became best friends in a matter of months.

The great thing is my son grew so much self-confidence having his best friend around. But even better, his friend, the former bully, completely stopped bothering the other kids as well. Having friends made him more sociable and friendly. They both gained in the process.

3.6 Submissiveness vs Shyness vs Introversion

Sometimes, we mix up introversion, submissiveness and shyness. There are three different things from a brain perspective. Submissiveness is about obedience and comes from the limbic brain. I've covered it before and won't go into it again here, but as a rule, it's fair to say it should be avoided. It's a burden.

Now, introversion, on the contrary, is a character trait and thus is in our new limbic brain. It's just something we are or not. There are introverts and extroverts, just like saying there are blondes and brunettes. I know our Occidental's society values more extroverts. However, when you look at Oriental societies, it's actually the contrary. Introversion is seen by them as a preferred character trait.

So, let's not stigmatize introversion. It's not a flaw. My son is an introvert as well. He doesn't mingle well and doesn't make new friends easily. Now, on the other hand, he's a great observer, has fantastic creativity and a strong analytical mind. Those things are linked. Every medal has two sides. And then comes shyness. Shyness is about fear of social fear. Somehow our brain has associated others, mostly strangers, authority figures and people of the opposite sex as a perceived danger. And then we freeze.

Now, it does lie in our genes to be wary of the unknown. It's a very successful survival mechanism. Recent research has shown, however, that the brain of shy people seems to take much longer to familiarize with new situations and people. The reptilian brain is putting us on red alert. So, now what I would say, talk to your kids, does he or she just like to be alone, which indicates introversion. Is he or she being picked upon, being bullied by other kids, which could indicate submissiveness? Or is he or she actually scared of all those people he or she doesn't know, which indicates shyness.

With introversion, my advice for you would be to build his or her self-confidence by focusing on what your child's good at. If you're too focused on the negative thing, what he or she is not good at, it's quite likely to be counterproductive. If you constantly repeat to our child that it's silly to be shy, he or she could end up thinking she's silly. I'm shy, so I'm silly. What do you think that does to their self-confidence?

If this is about bullying, I refer to a lecture on how I held my kid to overcome that, invite friends at home and yes, even to bully, friendship lurks around the corner, which is the best guarantee to stop the bullying.

So, what about shyness? The other is perceived as a threat. How can we overcome that? Remember that the reptilian brain is not where our reasoning lies. So, there is no need to try to rationally convince your kid. It just won't help. Look, we are all social beings. Connecting with others will help our children grow and they should do it and do it at their own pace. Luckily, we can guide them, facilitate things, show them how it's done.

Here are a couple of things that might help make it a home game for them. Invite same age friends over. Your home is familiar ground for your kids, so it's easier for him or her. Invite one at a time. Now, don't overwhelm your kid this way. They will be able to connect and develop a friendship. They will experience for themselves how the other isn't a threat, but a source of fun. Make the introductions just as you would introduce grownups to each other, introduce the kids to each other.

Hello Jamie, this is Nicholas. This is Jamie. Then just sit down with the two children and ask the other kids some questions, like if he has brothers or sisters, what is his favorite toy? Stuff like that. Instead of telling your kids it's easy to make friends, just show him how it's done, and then involve your kid. Wow. Jamie, you like Spider-Man? Nicholas does as well.

Another thing to do is to find a children's book about how the main character was able to overcome his or her shyness and tell it as a bedtime story. Your kid will be able to relate and have an example to follow. Whatever you do, don't make fun of his introversion or shiners in front of others. Never, ever. Don't ridicule him.

Don't even tease him about it. I mean, we'll talk about this later in the course. Just remember, for now, making fun of your kid, especially in public, is a no go.

But in the end, remember to give it some time as well, shyness is often a trait they outgrow. Once the brain learns that the other isn't a threat, shyness will just end the way the new neural pathway where others are associated with fun. New pathways will prevail over the old ones, where the others were synonym of danger. So, there you go. Submissiveness, introversion and shyness, each borne out of a different brain structure.

3.7 Why We Should Teach our Kid to Trust us

I would like to tell you about one of my favorite scientific studies is the marshmallow experiment of Walter Michel for that study, they told children they would get a marshmallow. The only thing they would have to do is wait for the scientists to leave the room, push a button. The scientist would come back, and they would receive the marshmallow easily. Now, here's the thing. They also told the child that if he or she would wait for the scientists to come back by himself, they would get two marshmallows.

What happens next is as cute as it gets. Some children don't even push the button and immediately eat the marshmallow. Some others tried to wait, but eventually pushed a button and with little voice claimed that "I only want one". But you can see on their face that somewhere they know that wasn't their best choice. Finally, some children were able to resist the temptation, wait the full 15 minutes and when the scientists come back, they get their second marshmallow. It would have been a cute hidden camera thing.

They did a follow up study 12 years later. What they found was astonishing. Those kids who successfully resisted the temptation 12 years earlier had better grades, were less likely to use drugs and even had a lower body mass index than those who hadn't resisted. Basically, the study revealed that the ability to delay gratification is a real factor of success in life. Now, the real question is, how do we get the ability to delay gratification?

Is it in our genes or is it something we learn? The answer came in a 2012 study conducted by Celeste Kids and some other researchers. As a follow up of the marshmallow study, the researchers found that delaying gratification is about more than willpower alone. The key lies in how our worldview was shaped in our early years. If we experienced our world as hostile and changing, our belief system will have encoded to benefit from things immediately, as they probably won't be around for long.

If the world was a stable and trustworthy place, we would have developed an unconscious belief system where it is worth doing something now and collect the fruits of our efforts later. Decades later, on a totally unconscious level, our decisions are still governed by this very strong belief system that determines a great deal about our lives. Now, what does this mean? That our whole lives are determined by the people who surrounded us when we were kids, when we basically couldn't decide a thing?

Well, it is always possible to rewire your brain. We can train ourselves or with the help of an outside person to teach our brain that it is OK to trust others, to trust the future. However, that's a whole other case altogether. It's so much easier to start off in life with the right script instead of rewriting, adhering to play. Help your children develop this one skill that will make a huge difference in their lives, to delay gratification through trusting future outcomes.

This way they will have the willpower to do their homework instead of watching TV, study for an exam, resist the temptation of being unfaithful to their partner, etc. Here's a recipe for a successful and fulfilling life. Not a guarantee, but a strong foundation that will favor it. So how do we do that? How do we build the skill of delaying gratification?

Some personalities are more inclined to make efforts, while others are more impulsive. So, not everyone starts off at the same level. Still, as with everything, it's something we can teach the brain. For you as a parent, this is what you can do when you promise something, deliver when they want something, make them earn it by making them clean up their room or something like that. When you warn them not to do something or there will be consequences to deliver the consequences. It has to be clear in their head that action means reaction.

If I do A, there will be B positive or negative. There will be consequences and consequences must be faced. It's very tempting to yield just to get rid of the tears and begging, however tempting. Don't let me put it quite dramatically. You are the guardian of the worldview of your children, a worldview that will govern the rest of their lives and lead them to success or failure.

Their future starts here. It started the day they were born.

3.8 Social Pain

Our species is not a peaceful one, and our Paleo limbic brain is mostly to blame for that. We fight, we mutilate, we kill evolution and survival isn't a joyride. Danger was everywhere. And even other humans could be a threat. So, this limbic amygdala, which is the center of fear and aggression in our brain, ended up playing a major role in the success of our species.

Interestingly enough, it also regulates parts of our social interaction & trust, the amygdala and the hypothalamus together decide who is friend or foe. The hypothalamus releases oxytocin, also known as the stress hormone or the bonding hormone. What many don't realize about oxytocin is that this hormone is also the one responsible for the famous "us versus them" behavior. It creates in-group dynamics and out-group dynamics. In other words, it's because of this hormone that we feel part of a group, being it family, friends, a sports club, a nationality.

And it's also because of this very same hormone that we will protect the group and exclude, even fight, those who are not part of our group. Those individuals who were successful in integrating into a group significantly augmented their chances of survival. That's why their genes were passed on from generation to generation and so on. And we today still have to deal with these remnants of our distant past. It's part of evolution. It's part of who we are, our very identity. That's why it feels so good to be part of a group. Our system gets flooded by oxytocin. It feels good. It feels safe.

Now, a part of adolescence is about that defining our own group, our own identity and fitting in. Adolescents need to develop these social skills which will help them create alliances in order to be successful later in life, create their own identity, their own social network. And as they create their own clan, we as parents, we get excluded. We're not part of their group anymore. Now, getting excluded from a group is a very dangerous thing to happen from an evolutionary point of view. It lowers our chances of survival when it happens. Evolution has made sure we would notice.

That's why there's an overlap of the neural pathways between physical pain and social pain. Yes, you got that right. Getting excluded from a group hurts. It hurts just as real as getting punched in the face or in the gut. It is true for our adolescents who will go the extra mile to fit in with their peers. It is true for my eight-year-old daughter who came home crying the other day because one of her good friends had been avoiding and ignoring her the whole day. And it is true for us, the parents, when our sons and daughters give us the cold shoulder and turn their attention to their friends rather than sharing with us what's on their minds. Sharpen your mind.

4.1 The Neo Limbic Brain

Our third brain structure is the neo limbic brain. I'm a huge fan of the neo limbic brain. It's a fascinating place, home to our deepest motivations and raw emotions. This is where our memory resides. Everything we experience in our lives will be recorded here. The good, the bad and the ugly. It's here where we are most of the time. I mean, this is a part of the brain that is usually running show.

It runs like an autopilot. It recognizes situations where we've already been through and immediately comes up with a set of standards operational procedures to deal with the situation at hand. It stores everything we've ever learned. It deals with everything from walking and talking, to driving and using a computer, to how to behave in public and all kinds of social codes. You can only imagine. It's highly efficient as it will use the minimum necessary attention span to carry out tasks, which frees up attention to do other things at the same time.

For example, let's say, driving and having a conversation with the person next to you, actually any routine occupation that lets you wander off with your mind. Here you will find all the contradictions and paradoxes of your complex personalities. We are wonderful beings capable of so much, yet limiting ourselves all the time. Basically, we can distinguish three layers of motivation.

The first layer is fixed, partly formed through our genes and partly from our environment. Once we are only three months old, it will remain the same for the rest of our lives. These motivations give us energy and joy. There are also intrinsic motivations with the NBA. We have identified different types of motivation, which lead to eight different personality types.

Now, every one of us has between two and four of these personalities. Sometimes they are very strong in presence. Sometimes, however, they get covered up and almost disappear underneath the other layers. The second layer isn't fixed. It will continuously evolve and has no age limit to do so. Here we will find our likes and dislikes. There are also extrinsic motivations. Extrinsic motivations aren't stable nor sustainable. They cost us energy and will fade if they don't meet with success.

Here we will find everything that our environment has given us, from our parents, brothers and sisters, our teachers and friends, to movies, music video games. Basically, this second layer is like a blueprint of the cultural influences we've been subject to. It pushes us to do what others expect from us. What is socially acceptable here lies also all our irritations, intolerances and prejudices.

The difference between the intrinsic and extrinsic motivations is basically the one with that little kid who has to clean his room in the first scenario. He'll do that and will actually enjoy the cleaning itself. Yes. Those gifts do exist. And the second scenario, he will be cleaning because Mummy told him to. Or because daddy promised something sweet. Will that same kid do his homework because he likes it, or because otherwise he might get punished?

And years later, will he go to law school because his dad is a lawyer. Or will he pursue his dream of working with, let's say, animals? And when the time comes to find a job, will he choose the one with a fat paycheck or the one where he loves the content. An important thing to know is that firstly, it will motivate you regardless of if you're great at doing what you do.

Extrinsic motivations, on the contrary, don't last. The motivation from a raise, if it's substantial enough, will last three to six months maximum. As a business owner, if you have to give your people a raise every six months, you'll be out of business in no time. The choice between a fat paycheck and a career you love is a no brainer from a motivational point of view. Still, a lot of people would go for the fat paycheck.

The society we live in pushes us to compete and win all the time. We're primed. We're biased. We're programmed to live a life that others intended for us. The real question, though, is underneath all that. What do you want? You, the real you, back to the three months old you, before everything else started to find a way into your limbic system. Why we should get happiness, fulfillment, joy. That's why. Otherwise, we'll just end up angry, frustrated and bitter. Faking to have a perfect life and being miserable inside.

OK, so much for intrinsic and extrinsic motivations, there is a third layer, though, a fascinating one. I'm talking about obsessions. I can hear you think, Oh, obsessions. I don't have those. That's nothing like me. Well, newsflash, I'm sorry to tell you we all have them. Not one wants to admit it, but many don't believe me. Fine. Be that way.

Remember the first time you fell in love? Remember the feeling? Remember how you just couldn't get enough of the other person you want to be together with all the time, calling and texting each other all the time, seeing the other person's face everywhere? Well, that, my friends, is what we call an obsession. And the fact that you think it doesn't apply to you is because you're not aware of them. An obsession is a passion that has gone over its tipping points. Behind it lies a compensation mechanism for a void in our life, when displaying obsessive behavior, and thinking all the time about something or someone.

Everything we do related to our obsession is just too much. We can't get enough of it and will never be satisfied. It's the root of addictions. It's more than the usual suspects of drugs and alcohol. Think about workaholism, shopaholics, gambling, stalking, fanaticism and extremism of all kinds. When they are not managed, obsessions can potentially ruin our lives and those of others.

But most of all, even when the obsession is mild. Due to its compulsive nature, it just enchains us into a life of servitude. Ever chasing that one thing that we can't get enough of? When obsessed with it, we are not free. So, to summarize our Neo limbic brain, it is our standby mode in which we operate most of the time and is also the home of our memories. Everything we've been through remains here. And most of all, the new Neo limbic brain is the heart of our motivations, of which we distinguish three layers. Our intrinsic motivations are extrinsic motivations and our obsessions. Sharpen your mind.

4.2 On Expectations

We just saw how compliments can affect our children because as we saw before, it's vital for a child to fit in. They're totally dependent on their parents. So, they'd better pick up on what is expected from them. Right. And they have mastered this. I mean, picking up on subtle clues to understand what is expected from them. And they will live up to our expectations even if we never even communicate this to them.

Look, what I'm going to share with you is one of the most surprising psychological effects around, but one that has been studied and corroborated so many times. It's been proven again and again and again. I know you will frown. I know I did, when I first heard about it. But it's spectacular. It's hard to believe. And yet it's been proven beyond any doubt, and it happens all the time everywhere. I want to talk to you about the Pygmalion effect.

The Pygmalion effect stage that other people will live up to our expectations based on what we think of them. In other words, how we think about others will influence how they perform. This has been studied repeatedly, especially within education and class settings. In one of those studies, in the beginning of the year, researchers would give a list of the new students to the teacher, telling them which ones were high potential and explicitly telling them not to show any favoritism during the year.

Now, at the end of the year, the high potential would systematically have the best grades of the class except that the list of high potentials list had been chosen randomly. It was completely accidental, and despite the teacher being told not to show any preferences, the kids would end up with the best grades. I know, shocking, right?

This is a pure self-fulfilling prophecy and has far reaching consequences because it works both ways, meaning negative expectations lead to negative outcomes as well. This one is called the GOLEM Effect. Now, know that there are hundreds and hundreds of studies out there, both with teachers and parents. And in 80 percent of these studies, the Pygmalion effect has been established. It's happening beyond any reasonable doubt, and we better be aware of it. It happens because even when we try to hide what we think about a child, there are always words or gestures or attitudes that will betray us.

And the kids are quick to pick up on them. They know understanding the Pygmalion effect and the Golem effect, of course, are crucial to understanding how stigmatization and stereotypes can boost or hold back children in their development. Well adults as well, but that's another story altogether. So, for example, there is this stereotype that Asians are good at math. I can assure you that there isn't such a thing as a math gene for Asians or girls aren't as good at science as boys.

Again, no such thing as a male science cheat. Then why is it that women are systematically underrepresented in science or certain neighborhoods and schools within them may be seen as no good or on the contrary, really good. Kids coming from those schools are seen as good or bad students even before they have the chance to prove anything. And the problem is not that much that we judge the book by its cover. That's human. That's how our brain works.

The problem is that the person in front of us, those children with so much potential, will end up conforming to what is expected from them. Now, this can be a good thing when we expect great things from them. But do you see how this can become a problem when expectations are low? OK, so now we've arrived at a crucial point within our relationship with our children. I get this question a lot. How demanding should we be for our kids?

And it's a legitimate question because on the one hand, if you put too much pressure on your kids and always ask more from them, you will raise insecure adults yearning for your recognition and leave them with serious attachment issues. Now, on the other hand, let them do whatever they want. Don't put any expectations on them, make their life as easy as possible. And what you get are spoiled brats who don't know how to stand up for themselves and go the extra mile. So no, how demanding should we be? Well, again, let me refer you back to Carol Dweck and the growth mindset. Let's not focus on results, but on attitude.

Be demanding on effort and forgiving on results. Teach our kids that working hard is the way to go and making errors is human and normal. And being lazy is a one-way ticket to failure. You know, the problem with being too demanding is that we create these expectations. And the message our kids get is that if they don't deliver the results, they're not worthy of our love. Of course, that's not true, but that's what their young brains get. It's a meritocracy. They must deserve our love.

I find that chilling, especially because they don't really have control over the outcome. Questions can be hard on the test, or the teacher has a bad day, or the kid was sick. I don't know. All kinds of stuff can happen. You know, when we as parents focus some effort on attitude, that's something they have full control over. If they put in the work, they know they're safe with us. It's not an endless bit of expectations that can never be filled. I know it's something they can own. So how high should we put the bar? How much effort is expected here? That's where Pygmalion comes in.

Discuss this with your kids, explain how much talent you see in them and how effort is the fertile ground where their talent will bloom. Set up rules you both agree upon. Be clear on your expectations. Let them set the bar, but challenge them, guide them in their growth and show them how it is done to exceed their own expectations. Give them a taste for hard-fought victories or even hard fights. Enjoying that, even without a victory, will set the stage for success in life.

Well, we'll talk more later about effort and grits, but it all starts here with how you look at your children and your expectations for them. Look at them with love, compassion, pride, and look beyond them. Look at what's in them, their potential, what they can become, because it's your way of looking at them, which will help them to be who they will become. Sharpen your mind.

4.3 On Punishments

We just saw how secondary personalities develop through our actions of punishment and reward. We will be shaping the behavior of our kids. Now, Skinner called this operant conditioning. Well, this process doesn't stop after childhood. It's a lifelong thing and will work with your partner as well. Now, if you want to punish and reward, there are a couple of rules you should apply for it to be effective immediately. The first one is never making a threat you will not act upon. Now, I understand in some situations we might get carried away and say things we don't really mean, but we must understand that this will damage our authority.

Jason, I swear to God, if you don't stop that immediately, I will put you up for adoption. And then Jason says, fine, put me up for adoption. Now, what are you going to do now? Big, scary parents. OK, I admit adoption sounds like the ultimate threat. Right? But what about having your kids making your life miserable in the car? Have you ever threatened to leave them on the side of the road and continue without them? Imagine your kid calling your bluff. Fine. Leave me. I don't want to be with you either. Then what? Your kid wins and you can only watch in despair.

Your authority crumbles in front of your very eyes. A couple of years ago, a few Japanese parents wanted to teach their kid a lesson that left the kids at the side of the road and drove off. The kid was seven. They drove like 500 meters and then came back. But guess what? The kid was gone. He had gone off to the nearby forest.

They didn't find him for another seven days, seven days. Lesson of this story? Don't threaten your kid to leave him or her unless you really plan on getting rid of your kid.

Sure. I take extreme examples to make my point, obviously. But this is true for the smallest of things as well. Take one to three, you count to three. And when you get to three, there's a punishment. It's a very effective method if you apply it right, because if you get to three and there's no punishment in no time, your kids will just ignore you. I know a mom who was using one, two, three and complaining the kids didn't listen.

Well, what she was doing was saying; 'kids, come on, let's go. One, two, three. Come on, let's go'. Yeah, no, that doesn't work. It only works when the kid knows there will be a consequence. So sure, you'll have to punish your kids once, twice, maybe three times. But I can guarantee you after that, your kids will jump and comply. So, what type of punishment are we talking about? It can go anywhere from a timeout to confiscating a toy or being grounded.

I'm against physical punishment. There are tons of studies showing how detrimental it is to hurt your child, to physically hurt them. You know, it's wrong on so many levels. Think about it for a second. What is the message we're giving them? Because you think you are bigger and stronger than them, you can hit them.? Is that the world view you want your child to have? The big ones can terrorize the smaller ones?

So, is it OK that your child hits smaller kids as well? And once he grows up, if it's a boy, is it OK to hit women to get what you want? No. Why not? Because they're adults. Oh, sure. You're only allowed to hit small kids who have no means to defend themselves in any way. That's not true. On a much more basic level, the question is, do you want your child to obey you because they love and respect you, or obey you because they fear you?

The best way to perform a punishment is as follows. First, the consequences must be clear and accepted. If you don't clean your room, you won't have Internet access for a week. They need to know what's at stake so they can make an educated decision about it. In an ideal world, you even discussed this with them and have them agree on the consequence. Look, I really don't like your swearing in this house. If you swear once more, what would be the consequence? Let them decide. Let them come up with a consequence.

You can always disagree if you feel they try to get away too easily once they've done the thing they weren't supposed to do. You need to apply the consequences discussed. You cannot let them off the hook. This is very important for you to understand from a brain perspective. Letting them get away, no punishment equals rewards. They get a dopamine shot, so if you don't punish them, you're actually rewarding them.

And what happens with behavior that's being rewarded? Exactly. It gets reinforced. In other words, they'll do it again because you just rewarded them for doing it. Look, the kids aren't stupid, they know well when they've done something wrong, when they did something, they weren't supposed to do, and forcing a consequence will help them develop a stable worldview and value system, which will be foundational for success later in life.

But more about that when we talk about the marshmallow study. For now, just know that you can't let them off the hook. It's not an option. Last thing I want to mention here, this process is very simple and rational. If you do this, there will be that. So, if this happens therefore, there shouldn't be drama involved, no yelling and screaming, you can just stay calm. You both determine the whole situation. "Look, buddy, we agreed you weren't going to make drawings on the wall anymore, and if you would do it again, there would be no more crayons for you and a time out to think this over. So, give me your crayons and go to your room."

Now, I know what you're thinking. That kid is going to make more drawings on your wall. Well, no, not if you sit down with him or her and explain calmly why it's important to you not to have these drawings on the wall and listen to your kid, why it's important to them to make those drawings. Then offer him or her an alternative, like readily available paper that he or she can use whenever they want to draw.

Now, this is all good and dandy when you can establish the rules before trespassing. But what happens when you're facing a crisis? Let's say, those Japanese parents and their seven-year-old who ended up one week surviving all alone in the woods? Well, the kid was being a total jerk and drove his parents crazy. Well, obviously, if done right, this situation never should have escalated in the first place. With the first warning, they should have established consequences and acted upon them.

Right. But let's say you're in the car. Your kids are having a fight in the backseat. They're driving you crazy. What do you do? Well, it has happened to me, maybe to you as well. What do you do? Well, we were just leaving for the holidays. We had a long road ahead of us and after like 20 minutes, the fighting started, I raised my voice. I started threatening. Nothing helps. I remember telling my wife I can just make a U-turn and drive home. You know, our holidays are over before they even start. And I was serious about it.

Well, that would have been a losing situation clearly for everyone involved, so I decided to do things differently, in a less confrontational way. I took the first exit and asked my son very calmly to get out of the car. We walked away, had him sit down and we talked. I explained to him how important these holidays were for me and how I needed his help in making them a success. We went back to the car, then I took my girl out, and did the same thing. We walked away, discussed the holidays and how I needed her help. We headed out and back to the car.

Guess what? We spent the rest of that day driving. It was a long road, and it was a blessing. Everything went fine. No more arguments. It was a fun road trip. Don't underestimate your kids. They get it, they know, treat them with love and respect, take time to talk to them to explain what is important to you and why they should care and help you.

Listen to them and their needs as well. Make them feel they're important to you because they are. You'll get way further and it will be a much more pleasant road than if you bully your way through their childhood, which works, of course, as well. But it costs more in - relationships and therapy afterwards when they're all grown up. Sharpen your mind.

4.4 Parenting Styles

Imagine this, your child is climbing a tree. It's the very first time he or she is climbing the tree. What do you do? Option one, you run to watch your kid and prohibit him or her from climbing any more. Option two, you let him or her climb. Both your arms are already open, ready to catch your kid if he or she falls down. Option three, you tell him or her to watch out because he or she might fall. Stay put when your kid eventually does hurt himself, you say, "I told you so." OK, that last one is a little bit harsh.

So, what do you do? Which one of these three options represents you? Now, I'm bringing this up because I know, as parents, we want the best for our kids. Ideally, we would like them to go through childhood without a scratch. But from a brain perspective, I mean, your child's brain learning process perspective, that wouldn't be advisable. Hear me out. You see, we should look at childhood as laboratory where our kids get a free pass to experiment without having to suffer the full consequences they would as an adult.

And the experimenting part is not optional. It's mandatory because it is at this time that our kids will acquire the necessary skills to be successful later in life. Those skills include things like how to get along with other people, how to solve problems, how to solve the fights, how to manage emotions, how to accept defeat, how to accept not getting what they want, how to overcome grief, how to deal with frustration, how to deal with emotional pain, and how to talk about all these things like emotions, pain, frustration and on.

It also gives them a chance of discovering what they like, discovering their talents, what they do that's enjoyable, any activity just for the sake of it, learning how to persevere when things get tougher, and then seeing for oneself that they get better at whatever it is they're working hard on. Also enjoying the work and learning the invaluable skill of delaying gratification, meaning doing the hard stuff now and reaping the rewards later. All these skills, all of them are crucial for a child to become an emotionally healthy, balanced individual, leading a successful, satisfying life.

When parents intervene the moment a problem arises, solving it for them, we basically deny them the opportunity to learn these skills for themselves. I know it's all based on good intentions. Don't get me wrong, I'm not judging here. I'm just looking at it from a broader perspective. And what I see is this by trying to make things easier and less painful for them in the short term, sincerely believing we're helping them.

Well, actually, we're not sure. In the short term we are. But in the long term, we're denying them the necessary experience, both positive and negative, that will help them grow and prepare for their life as an adult. And there is another aspect to this. When we jump in, whenever they face a challenge, the subconscious message we're sending them is as follows. You cannot do this alone. You need help. You're not capable. You need permission from someone else to do things you want to do. You see what's happening here? You see how all this is not helpful?

I know you're not saying that out loud. You're not even thinking that. But it is the message they're getting if repeated over and over and over again, it's what their brain will register and incorporate in their belief system, in their view of the world. And that is the kind of belief system that will hold them back their whole life long. It leads to what psychologists' call learned helplessness. In other words, we teach them to become helpless, to become dependent on others.

This is basically the exact opposite of what raising a child is all about, right? So, what should we do next? What is the right thing to do? How can we help them if we're not allowed to intervene? Right. Well, it's not like that either. Sure, we can intervene. Of course, we should help them. What I'm saying is, not right away. Jump in a few minutes. Something comes up, let them struggle for themselves. Let them try things out, let them get frustrated and get up and give them the opportunity to find a solution for themselves.

Then when they come to you for help, be there and guide them towards a solution. Show them how it's done this way. Next time they will be able to solve the problem by themselves. Now, let me share with you what is for me one of the most interesting theoretical frameworks regarding parenting. It is called the attachment theory. The central idea is simple. What kids need most are safety and exploration. Yes, both.

The idea behind it is the observation that the more secure a person feels at home, the more likely he or she is to venture out boldly to explore new things. This is true for adults, adolescents, kids and toddlers alike. Now the attachment theory, based on a mountain of research, explores the different scenarios based on different parenting styles and its impact over the course of a lifetime. The findings are actually quite interesting. It turns out that attachment, even at age one, correlates reasonably well with how people will do in school, how they will fare in life, and how they will develop relationships later in life.

Researchers could predict with 77 percent accuracy who would drop out of high school based on the quality of care given at forty-two months. That's three point five years old. The children who didn't drop out had developed a series of skills based on their unconscious worldview, who led them to build relationships with teachers and peers. The same skills would lead them to better romantic relationships and stronger teenage self-confidence levels, social involvement and social competence.

Now, I'm not saying that all our life is predetermined in that first year and that we have no control over it. Absolutely not. What does happen is that the relationship with our parents lays the foundation of how we look at the world, which will in turn shape our relationship with others. OK, first of all, let me be clear there. There is no one who writes parenting style from lenient to authoritarian.

That doesn't seem to influence the attachment too much.

We roughly see three types of relationships between parents and their children securely attached. Children have parents that are attuned to their desires and mirror their moods. They will calm them when they are anxious or sad. They will play with them when they are happy. By no means are they perfect. Of course not. I said before it's totally normal to screw up our parenting methods. These little beings will not break if we yell at them and lose our temper. If the overall pattern of care is reliable, coherent and predictable, then kids will feel secure in the presence of their parents.

Oxytocin will rush through the veins of parents and kids alike, and bonds will grow strong. Now, evidently less attached to children tend to be parents who are emotionally withdrawn and psychologically unavailable.

There is a lack of communication and affection between them. Now, what the child's brain learns is that it must take care of itself.

At first glance, one might think that's a good thing, right? When they get older, these kids are astonishingly independent and mature, at least at first sight. They fail to develop close relationships with other kids and adults alike. They suffer from higher levels of chronic anxiety and are unsure in social situations. Later in life, they withdraw before the other gets a chance to get close, as they haven't learned to deal with their own emotions and those of others.

The last category is the one of ambivalent or disorganized attachment patterns where parents are inconsistent. One moment they are all over their kids. The other moments they are nowhere to be seen. The kid's brain is not sure what to make of all this and fails to develop consistent working models. The result of this is when they grow up to be more fearful than others and have a hard time controlling their impulses. Higher rates of psychopathology have been observed during adolescence.

Now the good news is nothing is written in stone. First of all, these are tendencies and correlations and not direct causal effects. Second, we all have our genetic predispositions, and some kids are just way more resilient than others. And last but not least, we parents aren't the only influence in our kid's life. If somehow, we fail, they can still pick up a mentor or an aunt along the way who will help them bond and develop those healthy relationships.

The conclusion of this attachment theory is that we should aim to develop a strong, coherent bond with our kids to form a safe haven. They will venture forth and back exploring the world, feeling secure as they know they have us, their parents to fall back to if need be. So, if we go back to the beginning of this book with my example of climbing a tree, which one of the three options would you choose?

Don't allow them to climb. Allow them but be ready to catch them or warning them and then saying, "I told you so." The answer I would suggest is, none of the above. Let them climb, sure, if they feel they need to, and if they fall, well, be there to dry their tears and maybe share your own experience of that one time when you also fell, and it also hurt. Show them you can relate to their pain, show them you can show them it's normal to fall, that it's part of life, and that whatever happens, you are there for them if they need you. Sharpen your mind.

4.5 Your kid has personality!

It's almost as if the genes we will transmit to our children go through this random number generator. It's impossible to know beforehand how our child will be physically or personality-wise. However, our genes are not the only element. That's who our kids are. Who they will become is partly due to their unique combination of genes, but also to the environment in which they grow up.

The first selection will be done by our gene pool, but there is a second one. During the first three months of our lives, based on the early contact with our surroundings, our brain will select what is useful and what is not to eventually shape our primary personality driven by our intrinsic motivations. Remember that at that stage, the newborn babies' reptilian brain is extremely active.

Basically, it knows only four experiences; fleeing, fighting and freezing and a fourth one, which is a standby mode. When there is no perceived danger based on those first months, the brain will sublimate those four experiences and develop personality traits based on them. Fleeing will lead to a love for movement and change fighting to challenges in winning, freezing to sharing and caring and standby to contemplation and thinking.

OK, I can hear you think how much fleeing and fighting a newborn baby can do, how many experiences can he have? Yes, of course, all this takes place on a baby scale. It's about the baby having gases or reflux. It's about how much time he cries before someone comes and calms him. It's about noise and other stuff like that. Now, there are many more subtleties to this, however, I won't go into them and discuss it here.

What's important for now is that those personality traits inherited from our parents and activated through our first experiences as a newborn baby will form the cornerstone of who we are and what motivates us intrinsically. Now, look at your children. Can you see it? What is it that drives them? What's their intrinsic motivation? Everyone has one or two dominant ones. So, what is it? They like movement and change challenges in winning, sharing and caring or contemplation and thinking.

Once you have identified their primary motivation, you have to be aware of the following this what you just identified is their driving force in life. This is their endless source of energy and joy. It will give them purpose in life. It's what will define them. What should they study? What job should they take? What will make them happy, fulfilled. Their natural talents will be born from these primary motivations.

Unless... Unless we as parents let our own judgment and expectations get in the way. You see, we all have our dreams, we all have our struggles, and we all wish the best for our kids. The thing is, we are not our kids. They are not us. It's not because we want to become professional football players that our kid has that special talent, too. And you can change professional football player to a lawyer, doctor, etc.

And this is also true for little things of every day, forcing our child to do things or behave in a certain way just because we would have liked that to happen to us when we work is actually counterproductive. You see, on top of that first layer of primary intrinsic motivation comes the second one. That second layer is made of everything we learned from the people around us, it's a mix of education and life experiences. Basically, it's what the world expects us to be. It will push us to do things in a certain way.

However, it doesn't give us energy and joy. We do it because it pleases our parents, because we get good grades, because we have learned that if we behave like that, people will like us. The second layer is volatile. It doesn't give us energy, it costs energy, it fades when we don't get the rewards that come with that behavior. It's what we call extrinsic motivation.

Of course, there is the basic education of being polite and having good manners. I'm not arguing about that. There are the limbic limits that must be set and the new limbic conviviality rules that have to be learned. But ones beyond that, we shouldn't be too directive. By doing so, we risk burying those intrinsic motivations under a thick layer of social expectations. Now I have to say, it's not the end of the world.

You can become really good at something you don't particularly like. You can end up with a lot of success and social recognition, hey, maybe even become famous and rich. But in the end, there will always be those three things that will elude you. And those are fulfillment, joy, happiness and missing out on that. It's just a huge waste.

So, what can we do, what should we do? Well, as a parent, the best we can do is let our children experience life as much as possible, let them have new experiences, let them find out for themselves what they like, what they don't like. Give them this window of opportunity to explore the world themselves, but always within a fixed framework, a set of rules. Let them try things out.

Your kid wants to climb a tree, let them climb a tree. If they don't like it, you'll help them down. Don't let your fear as a parent stop them from climbing. They could fall. Sure, they could end up with dirty clothes. Yes, maybe some scratches, of course. So what? What if your kid, by climbing this tree, just took the first step of a road that will lead him to climb Mount Everest. Or maybe not, maybe he'll just love to hug trees because on an unconscious level, it will remind him of that blessed time as a kid when he climbed them.

Either way, why would you want to take that away from him? This is true for climbing trees and for everything else, the more restrictions, the more you cut off ways of letting the intrinsic personalities express themselves. But watch out. I'm not saying either that you should encourage them to do all kinds of things and cheer along the way. You might turn an intrinsic motivation into an extrinsic one. In other words, instead of doing something because he or she just enjoys doing, your kid could start doing it for the attention and approval he or she gets out of it.

So, in conclusion, don't restrict themselves too much, don't care too much, just let them be, let them experience the world and how they relate to it. Let them find out for themselves what they like and dislike, respect their choices, the difference and uniqueness. If they want to explore it further, facilitate it, give them information, give them options, let them decide. Don't impose, don't force them. You'll just get them confused without knowing what direction to choose in life. So let them be. Or as nature would say, let them become who they are.

4.6 Mindsets

Today, I want to talk to you about a whole discussion I have had with my wife. It was a couple of weeks ago and was during the exams of our kids. So, what happened basically is that while they were preparing for the exams, I started talking with the kids and I was saying, well, look, if you work hard, that's the most important thing. You can fail an exam still having worked hard enough. So actually, I'm less interested in how good your grades are and much more in how much work you put into.

My wife overheard that and then afterwards she came to me and said; "Did you actually say what I heard you say? What did you mean? What's the problem? You basically told them they could totally fail, and you were OK with that. So, like, yeah. And actually, I mean it. Hear me out. The thing is the exam is like a snapshot. It's one moment in time. I wasn't ready for that.

And I think and maybe because of stress, maybe they just think, well, maybe whatever, that they didn't perform well. Basically, that's the whole thing. It's a snapshot and it isn't a good reflection of their actual capabilities. So that's why if they work hard enough on it and even if they fail, it doesn't matter, because the fact that they worked on it, they develop their own agenda, even though they might not remember at the time of the exam.

In the end, it turned out OK, because they did the work and that's what really matters. I didn't agree with that. She went like, no, but exams are important. So basically, they start working and get good grades. And with your theory, they just don't care if they get good grades or not. They just do it. And whatever they're not focused on, that's not how it works.

I started explaining to her the difference between a fixed mindset and a growth mindset. This theory comes from Carol Dweck. Now, Carol Dweck is one of the leading psychologists worldwide. This woman is brilliant. And she was able to pinpoint some interesting words on a concept that is more broadly understood already. But the whole concept of the fixed and growth mindset is very helpful.

Basically, we were talking in a business environment, the difference between fixed mindset and growth mindset is the fixed mindset is where you focus on results. While the growth mindset, you're more process oriented. That's very interesting to look at, because some people have a misunderstanding of what the growth mindset means, some people will tell you need growth. Mindset is about capability of learning.

No, that's not what it is about. Of course, we're capable of learning, especially kids, right? Well, they adapt. They change, they grow. They learn, of course. But it's not about being capable of learning, the brain being capable of taking in more information. It's not about that with a fixed mindset. You look at results, your focus is on results. So, you want to get good grades. And in order to get good grades, you avoid taking risks.

You avoid getting out there and trying out new stuff. You stick to what you know. And that's why it's a fixed mindset now opposed to a growth mindset. That's the contrary. You're not focused on the results, on the actual grades you're getting, but you're focused on the process, on the learning itself, on experimenting, on trying out new things. And that's what the exciting part is all about with the growth mindset.

And it's not so much about getting good grades. It's about putting in the effort to get there and having to try some new ways to learn or to get results. And so, if you fail, that doesn't matter, because it was the work you put in there, the actual experimentation that was the most important and actually enjoying the process. We had this whole discussion and my wife said; "You know, if they fail their exams, that's going to be one for you."

OK, I'll take the risk by coming for that. So, the exams took place, and they came back, and they had mostly really good grades. A couple of them weren't good enough, but I mean, weren't what we were expecting or hoping they would get. But it wasn't at all the total fiasco my wife was expecting. The good news is with that little experiment of mine, we really could see that.

It doesn't matter if I had said focus on the results, it would have probably been more or less the same. But the difference is how they feel about it, because now suddenly you get to your exam, and you don't have the pressure to perform. You're much more relaxed because, you know, you did the work, so you don't have to be totally stressed out. If they get bad grades, they get home as well, and it doesn't affect your relationship or their relationship with you. It doesn't dependent on how good they score, how good grades they get.

No, it's about how much effort they put into working and into anything. And that is what is so important to me. But I'll get there in a moment. So, what I see here is a link as well with my business, because with a fixed mindset, oh my God, I would never, ever be doing what I'm doing here now. You have to understand my first nine months when I started the Neuro

Geeks, actually it wasn't even named a neuro geeks.

And I wasn't doing anything online. I was trying what I had always been doing before, giving workshops, giving coaching, etc. as the first nine months that I launched my business, I didn't get a single sale. I didn't get a single new client. So that was horrible. From a business point of view. However, the big difference here is that even though I didn't get results, people were asking me, "So how are you doing? What's up with you?" And explaining the brain working, blah, blah, blah, everything's fine. And usually ending with the words, "Now, if I can only find a way for people to pay for my work and to actually getting paid for the effort, I'm putting in there, that would be great."

But you see, I wasn't looking at the results. I was looking at the process. I really enjoy working with the content I was working with. I only had to find a way to monetize that. And then I went like, yeah, what can I lose? So, let's try something new, growth mindset, right. I tried something new. I went into online learning. I went into online teaching. I started creating my first online course, my very first months that I put that course online.

I made fifty-five dollars. Fifty-five dollars. I mean like fifty-five dollars. That was the first time in ten months I had made money, it was huge. That was great. And it was only fifty-five dollars. So of course, I wouldn't be able to make a living out of that. But that wasn't the important part here. It was the first time ever I was making money online and that was a blast. That was the best thing that ever happened to me, at least in those last ten months.

So, I'm like, yeah, let's go there. Let's do this more, because this might work. Now, if I had been result oriented with a fixed mindset, I would never, ever, first, have tried the whole online thing and segment. Would I have persevered because it took another six months before I had some more or less decent income and another year before I could live off that income.

So, with the fixed mindset after six months or after year, I would have given up easily. It's only thanks to the growth of mindset that you try out new things and that you're able to persevere and put in the work to get to success because overnight success doesn't exist or hardly does. There are months and years and sometimes decades of hard work behind it.

And if we can teach that to our kids to put into work and to enjoy the process, that's where they will find success later in life. But if you only have them focused on the results, immediate results. Oh, my God. So, I put the effort and I don't get the results. What are you going to do?

Hey, listen, I quit the whole bailout. They want specific. They want to do the work. They will stop. They will quit. That's it. They will quit.

Fast forward now. We're a couple of months later and my son will soon be turning twelve. So, we've started to look for schools for him and I've been visiting several of them. And that's been difficult because I was expecting so much from the big names. And when I went there, I was so disappointed. It was really turned off when I could see that there wasn't a real pedagogical project behind it and they were mostly surfing on that good name they've been having for years, sometimes decades.

And people put them there because they expect it's going to be a good school for their kids. Are you going to teach us anything or are we just going to sit here? That's not what I saw. That's absolutely not my experience here. What I could see in the big schools, the big Ivy League schools that I visited. And by the way, I don't live in the U.S. I live in Canada. My experience is only relevant to my location. However, it might be the same every place.

Please go and check it out. Don't jump to the conclusion because a college or school has a big name. It doesn't mean they have a valid, good pedagogical project behind it, because what I saw in the big schools was a fixed mindset. Basically, with those big schools are about is to prepare your kid to enter society and enter the whole rat race, and find a job, et cetera. But hardly anyone was talking about the importance of your kid to grow as a human being, to feel appreciated, to grow as a person, to be happy.

I don't think I heard the word happy in either of those big schools. What they were focusing on was, yeah, results and working hard. You're not working hard enough. I need results, but nothing for personal development. I was shocked. So, I visited several more schools. There was one. Oh, there was one that was good. I'm not going to give names here because that's not the whole point of this discussion.

But that was one school I found that was right. It didn't have a big name and it's a local school close to where I live. And they were talking about the growth mindset. We're talking about the importance of personal development, all those things that I was so missing in the previous audits, I really got charmed by the school.

So, what I found interesting here is that my whole trying to apply Carol Derek theory to the education of my kids was matched by what I heard in that school and at this school, I have to say yes, of course. And the way they tried to apply that is interesting. One way they would do that is by only giving personal grades, there wouldn't be any comparison with the other kids in a class or even school average or anything like that, meaning that they would be looking at the evolution of the child and compare him or her with his/her earlier grades.

The focus relies on that development there and not trying to compete or being better than the others. Another thing they were doing was that, sure, there are exams and sure there are tests. However, that wouldn't be the only thing that they would consider for giving points to the kids. So, 50 percent would be dictums. However, 50 percent of the grades would be based on the actual work the kid was doing during the year.

The tests, of course, but also the attitude in the class, the homework they would be doing, et cetera, et cetera. So, all that would be taken into account to evaluate the child's performance and not only the final results of the exam. The one thing I truly loved was how they said they were promoting independent critical thinking and immediately added to that that this was not the easy route.

I'm sorry. Too late. Excuse me. Do you know who I am? I have absolutely no idea. Good. The interesting part here is that in my course on leadership, I speak exactly about that. When you empower your people, when you make them critical, and you give them the opportunity to speak up, it's way more interesting, of course, and it empowers the individual. However, as a leader, it's not easy at all.

Applying that to a school setting is really brave. Imagine the teacher in front of 20 kids not agreeing with them on the point and having not the authority argument like, hey, I'm the boss here because I'm the teacher. You sit down, shut up and listen to what I say. No, you actually will have to convince them. And by making them critical thinkers and independent thinkers, your kids will be doing that even more.

So, they will speak up. They will disagree. It's a brave choice. And it is by far the most interesting choice from a development point of view for the kids. There were other things that they were trying to implement, but these were most important for me, the ones that stood out and made me seriously consider sending my kid there because the difference was so strong from the classical school and with a very good reputation.

But I was clearly into a fixed mindset where you would push the child to basically comply and become one of many others who will end up in the system. And then that smaller school, smaller meaning a name with a real pedagogical project for my kid daring to go the hard way, the less traveled roads. And by doing so, basically giving, in my opinion, the best chance to succeed. Why not? But if they really want to start their own projects, start their own organization, company, and stand up for what they believe in and try things out, and if it doesn't work, persevere.

I will be talking about grit in another episode. However, grit is by far the most important thing we can teach our kids in order for them to be successful later in life. And one way to do so is to give them this growth mindset, having them focus on the process rather than the results. Yeah. So, before you jump to conclusions and you see a big-name school, go there and listen to what they actually have to say.

What is their pedagogical project for your kids? Because just trying to do what everybody has always done, having them fit in through discipline and hard work, that won't cut it. That won't do, at least for me. Maybe that's what you want for your kid. I'd rather have them teach my kid how to be independent, how to enjoy the process of learning and persevering and focus on not so much the results, but the actual journey, the actual road traveled and having them enjoy that. Sharpen your mind.

4.7 On compliments

This one I get often. Is it good or bad to complement our kids? Some parents are concerned that complimenting too much will turn the kids into egotistical, lazy, couch loving materialistic tyrants or make them just weak. On the other hand, the concern is that if you don't compliment your kid, they will feel unloved, unappreciated, disconnected, won't develop their talents and will become distanced. So, what should we do as parents?

As always, it's about finding the right balance. And yes, there is a right way to do it. You see, whatever you're praising in your kid will reinforce his or her identity about that. For example, if you praise your child for working hard at school, it reinforces his identity as an industry soul. In this frame of mind, your child is willing to take on challenges and view mistakes as part of the process.

On the other hand, if you praise your child for being smart, he or she might end up believing that achievement is an inborn trait. And with that frame of mind, so your child will want to continue to appear smart, thus taking less risks and trying fewer challenging things because he or she don't want to make mistakes and appear stupid.

So, you see the huge importance of what we praise. Praising inborn traits such as beauty and intelligence can lead us to a sense of entitlement and develop dominance. The rules are simple. Don't focus on the activity, the effort, not on the results or the personality trait. So don't say while you're the best, say while you've worked hard, don't say, 'Oh, that's beautiful'. Say 'you really applied yourself'. Don't say 'you're such a smart kid'. Say 'you really do like to learn new things, don't you'?

Oh, and don't overdo it. Of course, we all need and like recognition. It's pure dopamine for the brain to hear someone praise us. The problem with it is that we get used to it fast and if we want the same dopamine. The rush will need stronger incentives over time. Not only will the Preying have less and less impact to trap here is that our kid can start liking the preying more than the activity itself.

This could lead to our kid turning away from something he or she was naturally good at just because he or she doesn't get the same dopamine rush anymore from our appraisal, when in fact the dopamine from the activity itself should have been sufficient. So do praise but praise the effort and don't overdo it.

4.8 Small Social Trauma's

A couple of years ago, I spent an afternoon at a friend's place. We have known each other since high school, and we've seen our kids grow. Our friendship is such that we can basically say everything to each other. That afternoon, his seven-year-old son was complaining about his little brother. I don't remember the exact details, but what I do remember was his dad's my friend's reaction.

Apparently, he likes to tease his kids, and just like that, he starts to sing this little song in front of me to his son about how he's just too weak, mentally inferior and stuff like that. Before he could add another verse, I'm brutally interrupted him. What the heck is your problem? He looked at me, apparently totally unaware of what he was doing and said, well, I'm only joking.

My son knows that. No, he should stop treating children like many adults. They do not have the same mental capacity to put things into perspective and are emotionally vulnerable. If there is only one thing you take away from this course and I mean, it's only one thing, I hope it will be this. I cannot stress this enough. Do not ever make your child feel ridiculed, especially in public. Public humiliation leaves scars, deep scars, and it could potentially affect your child's whole life in ways we cannot even foresee.

Why am I stating this so strongly? Let me explain to you the mechanism it has. Before the age of 17, a child doesn't have the PRE-FRONTAL maturity to put things into perspective, to be able to emotionally deal with the feelings of being ridiculed, even though the child is vulnerable, it is not defenseless. His brain will feel the intense emotional pain of the humiliation and will say never again. It will never again be put in such a situation.

What happens next is that the brain will, on a totally unconscious level, develop an avoidance and compensation mechanism. Let me explain this with a real-life example. Let's take Johnny. Johnny is an adorable young boy who one day during a family reunion sat down on his mommy's knees, gave her a big kiss and told her he loved her. The thing is, mummy had a tough day, a tough life, really, and love hasn't been working for her, so she pushes her son back and says, 'John Real man doesn't say things like that'.

Ouch. Johnny doesn't get it. He's hurt. He's confused. His brain learns fast, though it learns that expressing feelings is something very dangerous. Something that hurts. Since that day, Johnny is incapable of saying, I love you to a woman, he is a person who cannot express his feelings. Instead, he goes from one relationship to another.

Each time it becomes serious, it becomes time to talk about feelings he runs. But even though he flees at the same time, he yearns to connect emotionally, so he compensates instead of shutting live out. He goes from one relationship to another. He needs to feel loved, even though he himself is incapable of expressing it. And as you can see, this compensation mechanism is a highway to addictive behavior.

It is a rule of all kinds of addictions, workaholism, shopaholics, alcoholism, drugs, gambling, etc., etc. Another example let's call him Jimmy. Jimmy has learned a poem at school and during a family reunion, his proud parents tell him to recite it in front of everyone.

Unfortunately for Jimmy, his daddy has decided to boycott his seven-year-old son. He makes fun of him, interrupts him, makes him start all over again.

For little Jimmy, this is pure torture. His brain associates speaking in public with danger. So, years later, when his boss tells him to give presentations, Jim is totally panicking. He doesn't even remember the humiliation as it was pushed back into the subconscious as a defense mechanism. The avoiding and compensation mechanism is there, though, and so just to give himself a little courage, Jim starts drinking before his presentation, as he noticed it helps him to overcome his seemingly irrational fear.

To cut a long story short. Years later, Jimmy became an alcoholic, lost his job, his wife ran away, and he ended up in the streets. OK, I know, I know these are very dramatic examples. These are extremes, and most probably there were other factors at play as well. Still. Do you want to take a chance with your kids? I didn't think so. These public humiliations are what we call small social traumas. They include bullying and its new virtual equivalent cyber bullying from the age of 17 onwards.

We do not develop any new compensation mechanism anymore as our brain is able to deal with the unpleasant experience of public humiliation. The thing is, at 17, every one of us has had his share of small social traumas. We all have a compensation mechanism. Most of the time, we're not even aware of them, and most of the time they're not really harmful.

Still, such a small social trauma which is completely harmless from an adult point of view has the potential to do a lot of damage in a child's experience. Not every time, of course. It all depends on how the child experiences the humiliation. But still, why take any chances?

Just don't do it. Life is already challenging enough. There's really no point in carrying extra weight.

5.1 The Prefrontal Brain

Last but far from least comes the Prefrontal brain. This one is a marvel of evolution. It makes us humans unique as no other living being has this brain structure the way we have it. Because let's face it, everything we've seen so far, all three brain structures are widespread in the animal kingdom. The reptilian and paleo limbic mode are so basic that using them puts us in a state where we have no connection anymore with our logical thinking abilities.

On the other hand, it is true that in the new limbic lies the essence of who we are as individuals with our memories and motivations.

Still, that doesn't make us human. Anyone who has a dog or a cat at home will be able to testify that those animals have their own character traits, likes, dislikes and motivations. So, it is the prefrontal brain that makes us human. Not so much the fact of having one as some of the more evolved mammals also have a prefrontal brain.

I'm thinking here, for example, dolphins, dogs, elephants and the other great apes the size of their prefrontal brain is actually the normal size. Ours is just ridiculously huge. It's almost as if it weighs a pint and it is this oversized Prefrontal brain that makes us truly human. How?

Well, remember our caveman from the reptilian brain, the one who was being hunted down by a pack of wolves? Yes, him. Well, if you compare him with a cave bear, there is one thing that distinguishes both. Even though generations of cave bears lived for thousands of years and caves, never has one of them thought about decorating the place. I mean, putting a little paint on the walls, drawing some wild animals is going to hand.

OK, ok, sure. Bears can't paint. So, what about the Sea Lion? Why haven't they used it to carve some nice patterns or maybe just a signature dive at the entrance to the cave. Was this why prefrontal brain size? That's why this Prefrontal brain works like a supercomputer on a totally unconscious level, drawing conclusions from all the different sensorial inputs it gets, creating innovative combinations to come up with new ways to deal with the situation at hand.

This way, the Prefrontal brain is a champion of adaptation and creativity, especially suited for a known and complex situation. As we saw before, the new limbic brain works as an autopilot dealing with the world as we know it. It is the home of all our little habits and routines which make us function very efficiently in our daily lives.

The prefrontal brain is the one dealing with new and complex situations. Let me correct that the prefrontal brain should be the one dealing with new and complex situations because, no, it's not always the case. Let me give you a couple of examples of automatic mode when adaptive mode would have made a huge difference to a publishing firm, turn down J.K. Rowling's first Harry Potter book.

Decca Records turned down the Beatles in 1962. The Titanic. I think there's a world market for maybe five computers, said the IBM chairman in 1943. Who the hell wants to hear actors talk that came from Warner Brothers in 1927 and Atari and HP turning down Steve Jobs idea of a personal computer? Now, I could go on like this for hours whenever someone thought of something new.

There have always been others unable to see further than what currently is, failing to see what could be. They stayed stuck in their limbic mode when what they should have done is switch to their Prefrontal brain. Now, the point I'm trying to make is that when we use our limbic brain, we're not able to see further than what we already know our existing experiences, hence the turning down of big opportunities.

When we must make decisions on new things, we should switch to our Prefrontal brain. This one enables us to adapt to change and deal with complex decision making. It doesn't ensure we'll make the right decision, nor does it mean we'll agree with any change just for the sake of adaptation. No, no. It only means we'll use all our knowledge and creativity to be able to see a possible future and then decide, yes or no. This contrasts with the limbic brain where we'll just reject it, because it has never worked before.

So, the reaction of Warner Brothers, who wants to hear actors thought it's a very good example of this at this point in time in 1927, all movies were mute. His limbic brain couldn't imagine anything else. His prefrontal brain would have been able to and maybe he still would have decided not to go for it, maybe because of financial reasons, high investments, but not because he couldn't imagine people not wanting to hear people talk.

Ditto with the IBM chairman stating there was a world market of maybe five computers, his limbic brain couldn't project a world with computers no larger than a book and much more capacity than at that time. Of course, not all change is good, neither is old resistance bad using our prefrontal brain when we need to help, since taking into account all the available information and taking the best possible decision based on that.

Our prefrontal brain is also home to our creativity, intuition, spirituality, but also, our adaptability. An indicator that our prefrontal brain is active is our emotions. We feel calm, serene and in full control. We are on top of our game. This is the true land of possibility right there behind our full head of prefrontal cortex, the marvel of evolution.

So, to summarize the Prefrontal brain, this is the part of our brain which should switch on whenever we face a complex situation, or we need to adapt to new circumstances. Unfortunately, often we don't, which leads to resistance to change and bad decision making. Sharpen your mind.

5.2 Two tricks to stay calm

When raising kids, it's as much about kids as it is about parents. In an ideal world we, the caregivers, are mature self-controlled individuals who know what's best for our kids and remain calm in the face of adversity. Yeah, right. In the real world there are a zillion of things influencing our state of mind from lack of sleep over work, stress to form schedules that need to be respected and kids who don't want to cooperate.

So yes, there will be times that you'll be about to lose it. Let me give you two little tricks that will help you remain calm when your only wish is to put your kids up for adoption. The first one is by activating your Prefrontal brain and imagining yourself 10 years from now looking back at this day, at this very moment. What will be your thoughts about this very moment 10 years from now?

You'll quickly realize that there is a 95 percent possibility that you won't even remember this very moment. And for the five remaining percent that you will remember you'll probably end up laughing about it. So, is it worth it to get all upset about it? The second trick is even easier than the first one. Just look at the situation and imagine how it could have been worse and that as a matter of fact you're well off by making your brain come up with alternative scenarios to what's currently happening.

You'll automatically activate that prefrontal brain of yours. This in turn will switch off the amygdala. Who at this very moment has labeled your kids as a threat that needs to be dealt with. The Prefrontal brain will re-establish balance by putting things into perspective. What are some other tricks to remain calm? There are more than 40 different ways to deal with stress. If you need some inspiration, make sure to find a stress relief course.

5.3 The Mozart Effect

Classical music lovers around the world rejoiced when they first heard about what became known as the Mozart effect. The story went on that if you would let your baby child listen to classical music, it would give him or her a higher I.Q. Some went as far to put headphones on their belly so their unborn child could already benefit from this amazing discovery. Amazing. Yes, but unfortunately not true.

Now, to be fair, there has been a study in the early 90s that saw a temporary enhancement of the spatial reasoning, which didn't exceed 15 minutes after being exposed to classical music. The study wasn't about kids, and it wasn't about IQ. Still, somehow some articles were written, some links were made, and the myth was born. Your research didn't find any link between children, IQ and classical music or any other type of music, for that matter.

Now, of course, that doesn't mean you shouldn't let your kids listen to classical music if they enjoy it. Great. What you will get is traditional enjoyment, arousal, which they would get anyway with any other type of music or listening activity that they enjoy. Sharpen your mind.

5.4 On Learning

A lot of parents are concerned about school and the results of their kids, you might be one of them unless your kid gets straight A's. Having said that, it's important to note that perfection isn't required nor particularly desirable. You see, if your kid is smart enough to get in a good school, he or she will be smart enough to excel. There's no correlation between accumulating large wealth and high IQ.

Now, of course, some Americans who won the Nobel Prize in chemistry and medicine did go to Harvard and MIT, but they were a minority. It was enough that they went to good schools, most, however, went to schools unknown to the general public. Now, of course, your ambition for your kid might be slightly different than a Nobel Prize. Well, here again, people with high IQ do not have better relationships and better marriages.

They are not better at raising their children. IQ predicts only about four percent variance in job performance. The parents and community have a greater effect on achievement than school. So how can we help our kids become smart enough and help them get into those good schools? From Green's perspective, when it comes to teaching and learning, there are two processes that are most effective.

The first one is to force your kid to make mistakes. I know it doesn't sound very nice, but it's highly effective. Millions of years of evolution have embedded a mechanism in our brain where we learn quickly out of our mistakes to get a higher chance of survival. Now, in the context of school, the pain of getting things wrong and the effort required to overcome error creates an emotional experience that helps burn things into the mind.

The second process is the act of retrieving knowledge. You see, when you learn something new, we create a new pathway in our brain. The more we use this pathway, the stronger it becomes. So, retrieving information strengthens the relevant networks in the brain. So, to resume when your kid comes home with assignments or must prepare for a test, let him or her study first. Once they're done, take some time to go over it with them, ask them questions.

That's their knowledge. Every time they answer, they strengthened neural path towards that specific piece of information. If they don't have the answer, don't hold them. Don't make it easy on them. Have them fail with you in this safe environment, it's better for them to fail with you than in front of all their friends in class. So have them repeat the parts they're weaker at over and over.

Some studies suggest that repeating something like six times will make it stick. Another thing, we retain information better when we alternate settings, so it does them in the living room, then go to the kitchen and to the garden, whatever. Once your kids grow up, help them by creating an atmosphere, an environment that favors studying.

You see, it is far better to go over material for a little bit repetitively on five consecutive nights than it is to cram in one long session the night before the exam. Oh, and one last thing. Sleep, sleep improves memory by at least 15 percent, make sure your kids and teenagers get enough of it. It will improve their memory, but also their general mood and immunity system.

Neuro Geeks

5.5 Adolescence

A lot of parents dread the adolescence of their children. There are so many wild stories out there and they go from slamming of doors to runaways from lack of respect to reckless behavior. Sometimes it seems like your loving, friendly child turned into this weird alien you're unable to connect with anymore. You probably remember how I said that our brain is fully mature at the age of 24.

Jumping to conclusions, one might think that's the explanation for everything. Their brain isn't working properly yet, suggesting they somehow became mentally impaired during adolescence. Well, that's not at all what's happening. You see, from the age of 12 onwards, our brain undergoes extensive remodeling. You can compare it to a network of wiring, upgrade the physical changes moving in slow ways from the brain's rear to its front, from areas that look after older and more behavioral basic functions such as vision and movement, to the more complex thinking areas.

However, do not underestimate the adolescent brain. It turns out the process of upgrading the brain isn't just a transition period between childhood and adulthood. It does serve a particular purpose. And as such, adolescence is a highly functional, adaptive period. So first, when your adolescent yells at you, 'I'm not a kid anymore', well, he or she is right. A child's brain is different from an adolescent brain, which is again different from an adult brain.

The first thing for you as a parent to understand is that your kid is not a kid anymore. The sooner you accept that, the easier it will be. True, they are not adults yet, but they are definitely not children. So, stop acting as if they were. The situation has changed. You are in a different game now and the rules of the parenting game have evolved.

I know for some of us this may be emotionally difficult to accept. And yes, for some of us our child will always be our baby. Having said that, I would like you to think about your role as a parent. There's no easy way to say this. So let me put it bluntly. Are your children there to attend to your emotional needs? Are you there to attend to theirs?

If you choose the first one, those adolescent years will be a tough ride both for you and your teenager. If you choose the latter, you're still in for a ride. But with the right Prefrontal attitude, you'll be able to become that safe haven, where your "almost adults" will gladly come home to for guidance and advice when they need, even though most of the time it will look like they just use you and your home for sleep and food.

And for some, there is a little bit of both. You see, there's a reason why your child is going through all those changes. There's a reason why if you hang on to the past, things will turn ugly. The process that is taking place is something of old times, the ancient Romans, Greeks and even Mesopotamians already complained about their use and how they lacked respect and stuff like that. Adolescence is not a cultural thing.

It's in our genes. It's human nature. And it's there for a reason. And that reason is to produce a creature optimally primed to leave a safe home and move into unfamiliar territory as a species. It is written in our DNA that we will leave our parents and start our own home. In order to do so, we need to overcome the fear of leaving something safe and warm and develop skills to survive in a complex and potentially dangerous world.

We will need to learn fast. We will have to take risks and we will need to find new allies. And that is exactly what our brain is doing. Let's have a look at what is going on in that alien brain of our teenager. We all know and probably remember of those raging hormones, right? Well, there are two of them that are of particular interest to us. The upgrading, adolescent brain becomes very sensitive to dopamine and oxytocin. Let's start with dopamine.

Dopamine is a neurotransmitter that primes and fires the reward circuits and aids and learning patterns and making decisions. This explains the extraordinary speed of learning displayed by teenagers. It also explains how success and defeat are met with extreme emotions. It also explains the love of the thrill, always on the lookout for something new, something exciting, unusual, the unexpected.

To get this one right, sensation shouldn't be mixed up with impulsivity. You can carefully plan something sensational like bungee jumping, for example. Impulsivity generally drops throughout life, starting at about age 10. Love the thrill, however, peaks at around the age of 15.

Oxytocin is not a neural hormone. This one is responsible for bonding and social cohesion. It explains why it becomes such an important factor during adolescence. Oxytocin has a dark side, though. It creates a feeling of us versus them, even though this gives an evolutionary advantage in terms of survival, it's also responsible for your teenager's hostility towards you.

Now, combining both hormones, what you get is youngsters who are very active, socially sensitive to peer pressure, always on the lookout to meet new people and share their stuff with them. Dopamine will push the youngsters from roughly 15 to 25 years of age towards risk taking, especially when other adolescents are around. The funny part is adolescents use the same basic cognitive strategies that adults do, and they usually reason their way through problems just as well as adults.

They think, as well as adults and recognize risk just as well. However, teens take more risks not because they don't understand the dangers, but because they weigh risk versus rewards differently. The dopamine makes the reward look better. It gives more way to the payoff. Now, from an adult's point of view, what we see is the bad influence of friends. When they're together, they only do stupid things from an evolutionary point of view. They are teaming up and preparing themselves to enter the big world.

The moment they do, they will have to change, to adapt, try out new things in order to make it.

And that's exactly what all this experimenting and crazy stuff does. I know from the outside, it doesn't look good. It actually looks like they have never been less ready to face the world on their own. But that's because we're looking at the outcomes and not the attitude driving the experience. They are about to conquer the world. And to do that, you need guts. You need audacity. While on a new path, have people follow you and support you. You need to be fearless. You need to find your uniqueness, your unique path that will lead you to a life worth living.

And that's exactly what the adolescent brain, with all its excess and drama and experimentation, is doing. Preparing the adolescent to spread its wings and fly. It's going to be legendary. So where does that leave us, the parents? It's definitely not something we can stop from going to happen, whether we like it or not. However, that doesn't mean we should let them do whatever they feel like in the name of evolution or something like that.

Adolescents need rules. They still need a framework, but one that is flexible and evolving. Just as they grow and evolve, they will gradually need more independence in order to answer their social needs. Refuse it and you will become the enemy. As a limbic brain is quite active during adolescence. It can turn into a pure territorial confrontation. When your child is five, it's easy to win the big battle when your child is 15, it's a different game.

Studies showed that when parents engage and guide their teens with light but steady hands staying connected but allowing independence, their kids generally do much better in life. The best way to deal with it is to put down rules, even in writing, if necessary, and the consequences of transgression. The rules must be clear and understood. However, you're not imposing the rules. You negotiate with them. Yes, you heard that. Well, negotiating.

Why? Because you're not the enemy. Remember that people support a world they helped create. You need their cooperation. So, sit down, explain to them what you deem fair. This can cover pocket money, how often they go out and what time they should be home, when to call and stuff like that. If they agree, fine. If they don't listen to their point of view, ask them why and try to find common ground. Do this exercise every six months.

If they're not happy with the outcome, you can always explain that they will have a new shot at convincing you in six months' time. Regarding those rules, I would like to recommend something regarding sleeping patterns. Sleep deprivation leads to irritability, depression, lack of attention and increases impulsive behavior. In other words, make sure your teenager sleeps enough. Adequate sleep is central to physical and emotional health. Don't let them stay up late during weekdays. Make sure there is a sleeping rhythm routine.

It will make your daily life much more pleasant. The parts of the prefrontal cortex develop at varying rates. The parts associated with cognitive control, including planning ahead, controlling impulses and regulating emotions are last to mature. So, if your teen's behavior upsets you or worries you, you know that one's prefrontal area is getting their upgrade, things will get back to normal.

However, there is a cost to that. Once the upgrades, the wiring is done, the brain loses flexibility. This is best shown with language acquisition, the brain's language center, one of the first to mature at around age 13. This maturity consolidates the gains but makes further acquisitions such as a second or third language much harder to come by. It's the same with the prefrontal cortex.

Reaching maturity ensures a higher speed, and we get better at balancing impulse, desire, goals, self-interest, rules, ethics generating behavior that is more complex and sometimes at least more sensible. The downside, however, is that we will never again be able to learn something up to the level of it becoming second nature, being used in sports, language, music or any other skill.

We will still be able to learn but will never again be able to have a native level at anything new we learn. Just have a look at how quickly adolescents pick up new technologies. Now look at how long it took you to reach their proficiency. Oh, you haven't. You mean they learned it faster and better than you ever could. So now how do you think teenagers look at the adult's brain, huh? Who seems mentally impaired now?

5.6 Screen Time

Let's talk now about a topic which most parents seem to struggle with, which is screen time, and I'm talking everything here, you know, smartphones, tablets, TV, video games, Internet, everything. So the latest figures show is that teens spend an average seven hours and 22 minutes a day in front of screens, and that is not including homework, seven hours.

And that's an average, you know, meaning some are consuming way more than that. If you look at kids between eight and twelve, we're talking about an average of four, four hours and 45 minutes. Younger children average over three hours a day. Again, this means some kids consume way more. So, what about your kids? When you look at these averages, are they below that level or above?

And remember, we're talking about everything here from TV to their smartphone. And whatever your estimates, reality is probably way higher anyway. So, what does it mean? And should we be worried? I've heard countless arguments, pros and cons, from the most convincing one being that technology is all around us and that we should educate our children to be fluent in its use because otherwise they'll probably end up as social outcasts with their peers.

Peer pressure. There you go. I felt it strongly when my kids were merely babies. My wife and I decided to avoid screens for our kids as much as possible when we discussed the topic with other parents. We felt like social outcasts, you know, some kind of extremists. It was weird. And now my oldest son will soon go to middle school and there's a whole smartphone discussion again. And we feel the pressure again to buy our kids their own smartphone.

Well. Ever since we had those first discussions about screentime, I decided to dive deep into this matter and see what science says and ever since then, I've been on the lookout for new studies and developments. So, the American Academy of Pediatrics recommends limiting the screen time for kids to less than one or two hours per day, depending on age. Of course, and for kids under the age of two, get none. Some pediatricians and neuroscientists even advise banning screens completely before the age of three.

So why do we do this? Why takes such measures? How bad can it be? Right. Well, I was about to give you a whole sum of the negative impacts on the brain, including brain matter, atrophy, loss of white matter, integrity, reduced cortical thickness and impaired cognitive function. All these are true and scientifically proven and scary as it sounds. What does it really mean?

Well, in short, excessive screen time impairs the structure and functioning of the brain. Last year, new studies came out about how toddlers who had excessive screen time had slower cognitive development and language acquisition. The link between screen time and obesity in kids was established a long time ago. There are also studies linking adolescents and screen time to increased anxiety and depression. You know, I can go on like that, you know.

But let me try to explain this in another way. Digital technology does not only consume attention, but it also shapes the brain. All these devices and apps are designed to grab our attention and not let it go. They are cleverly designed to tap right into our reward system. We get instant little kicks of dopamine. Every time we reach a new level of a game, we defeat an enemy boss. We watch a funny video on YouTube or even when we hear the little beeping sound of a new message.

Dopamine is all about instant gratification. It's about here and now and feeding our kids brain levels of dopamine that they would never get in an On-Screen environment is a recipe for disaster with an average of seven hours of high dopamine screentime. The rest of the day looks pretty dull and boring, you know. That part of the day when they ought to be at school and learning the skills and acquiring the fundamentals that will help them become successful individuals in their later life?

Yeah, well, with the constant thrill-seeking behavior, the kid's brain is on the lookout for the next dopamine shot, which means that kids become increasingly distracted and won't be able to focus. And if you can't focus, you can't learn. The instant gratification that children get from their screens is in direct contradiction with the patience and grit one needs to be successful in life.

Yes, Grit's, I've talked about it before. Remember the marshmallow experiment of Walter Mishel, it all comes down to those 30 years and how we are able to say no to temptation. The more we can resist, the stronger we will stand later in life. Unfortunately, it doesn't stop here. The time our kids spend in front of a screen, they are not spending developing other necessary skills.

Small kids, toddlers who are spending too much time in front of a screen are developing to define what skills they would otherwise be playing with clay, scissors, coloring, drawing, etc. You might already have seen a toddler trying to change the page of a book or magazine by swiping it. Well, as funny as it seems, it's a clear warning that screentime is off balance and there is more. What can we say about the impact of screen time on socialization, emotional intelligence and psychological well-being?

One of the greatest developments in the last decades in the field of psychology is a surge of positive outlook, instead of looking to understand what was wrong with us. This branch of psychology seems to understand what makes us happy. Well, the answers found were disturbingly simple and old, pointing in the same direction as the other. Yes, we are social beings. It's the core of who we are as a species and is the reason why we were able to say farewell and rise against all odds to dominate this planet.

We find meaning, consolation, hope and happiness. When we share our time on this earth with the people we care about, it fills us. It completes us. It turns us into healthy and balanced individuals. Now, look at screen time again. What happens? Kids alone in their room playing games. Even when they are together, they are alone. Due to our limited attention span, we can only focus on one thing at a time. And screen witness.

OK, one more, just in case it wasn't already bad enough, sleep deprivation, the excitement of the dopamine rush is obviously not compatible with the quiet and calm we need to find sleep now. Devices increasingly use these blue light-led screens, which also disrupts melatonin, and rhythms to keep us from falling into Morpheus' arms. Now, if there is one thing that every parent knows is that a child who lacks sleep will become cranky, irritable, moody, won't be able to focus, let alone learn.

We've spoken about sleep before extensively. And of course, this is basic but crucial. Now, of course, all these things won't happen if you let your child use these devices from time to time with moderation. And when visiting friends or family, your 12-month-old baby ends up in front of the TV watching the Teletubbies. It won't cause brain damage either.

It's about patterns, repetition, daily reinforcement of stimulus, which end up altering the brain. And of course, a Skype conversation with your aunt is not the same as a game of fortnights where you basically, have to kill everybody else to win the game. So, I guess it all comes down to what foundation we want to give our children. Allowing excessive screen time won't turn them blind or crazy. As always, it's much more subtle than that and has consequences in the long run.

It's about patterns and repetition. It's about daily habits. And the rules here are very simple. The lesser, the better. Now, I'm not saying to totally shut down screentime. It's fun, it's entertaining and used with moderation. It's a source of lots of fun and excitement. But when consumed in excess, screen time is counterproductive to laying the foundations that will turn our children into the bright young men and women we hope they one day will become.

My kids, well, they didn't get any screen time before the age of four from four to eight, they could only watch half an hour and this only during the weekends from eight onwards. This was upgraded to one hour on the weekend, meaning one hour on Friday after school, one hour on Saturday and one hour on Sundays. Once they reach 12, well, we'll re-evaluate and plan on giving some more screen time.

And of course, there are exceptions. For example, when we go to the cinema and watch a film together. Right. At first, most of our friends were shocked. Nowadays, most of them complain about how they're like kids. We're talking 10-year-olds here are already addicted to their screens. Remember dopamine? And they want to know our secret. How do we do it? Well, that's actually easy. We never let it go out of hand in the first place. It's easy to keep control that way.

You know, it's like a discussion I had with my son. I told him I was doing this experiment and stopped drinking alcohol for 100 days. He looked at me and said, well, why not a year? And I said, one year is a long time. It's hard. And he said, well, I haven't drunk alcohol for 11 years. It's not that hard, huh? He cracks me up sometimes. But actually, that's the whole point. You see, it's so much easier to quit when you haven't started.

The same is true with screentime. Keep it under control from the start and it will be way easier down the road because of the high dopamine levels. Some people have compared screen time with alcohol. Of course, that's not technically correct, as alcohol has other negative effects on the brain, as we've discussed before. But I do agree on the fact that screen time is a digital drug and we as adults have the responsibility to help our children consume it in a responsible way. Sharpen your mind.

5.7 Grit

OK, we need to talk about grids. Call it what you want, perseverance, endurance, willpower, the capacity to continue when things get tough. Grit is the single most important element that will determine if your son or daughter will have a successful life. Whatever definition you give to success, it can be material financially. It can be a career, starting a business. It can be relational. Having a happy and fulfilling relationship and raising their kids.

It can be all of them combined or even something completely different, like winning the Nobel Prize or a gold medal at the Olympics.

Whatever your definition of success, the single most important predictor of that success will be grit, not IQ. I said it before, IQ correlates poorly with a career or even winning Nobel Prizes. The average for the Nobel Peace Prize is one hundred twenty-one. Well, I have a hierarchy in that. I mean, they can always call me, but it's not likely to happen.

You need something else, something else, than IQ to make it. And that thing is Grit. Now, grit is closely linked to several other elements we've discussed in this book. Remember the marshmallow test and delayed gratification. Remember the growth mindset and how to focus on process rather than outcome. Remember learned helplessness and how they need to learn for themselves how to overcome challenges, right? Well, it's all interrelated and it all leads to higher grades.

When our children develop grit, it's not just about toughening up. It builds their character and helps them prepare for lifestyle changes. You get bad grades at school. What do you do? Change studies or try harder? Your boss is critical of you. What do you do, change jobs or try harder? Your relationship is rocky. Your partner wants to give up. What do you do?

You see where I'm going, right? You can do this for everything. Whenever an obstacle emerges, how will you respond? Will you quit or try again? Do things differently. Try another angle. Search for a solution. Do you see how that helps in everything, in more stable relationships, a better career at school, in sports and pretty much everything? The interesting part is our kids need to fail to get there. They need to learn from those failures. It's the growth mindset, right?

They need to bite the dust, get back up and go along with the bitter taste of defeat still in their mouth. OK, that was maybe overly dramatic, the bitter taste of defeat still in their mouth. No, as explained before, there's an easier way to do so. Love the process and see every challenge and this as an opportunity, because what happens if they don't learn how to taste the bitterness? Why do I get that stuff? What happens is simple.

The moment a real challenge arises when you need to go the extra mile, they will give up looking for excuses rather than solutions. They will point fingers at everything and everyone except themselves. I've seen this happen so many times around me. Parents work hard and make it. They spoil their kids. Kids grow no spine and become useless adults. It's a classic. It happens everywhere and all the time. So how do we help our kids develop this grit, discipline and authority?

The answer we talked about was the Pygmalion effect. Be demanding. Raise the bar. But how high should we raise our bar? Grit is linked to adversity in childhood. Kids who had a tougher time developed it, but not always. Sometimes they get crushed, and you get the opposite. Some kids who faced adversity in childhood develop grit. Yes. Some of them, however, develop what scientists call learned helplessness. That same learned helplessness, or at least a close version of it, where they give up, look for excuses rather than solutions.

They point fingers at everything and everyone except themselves. So, what's the difference between the adversity that leads to grids and the one that leads to learned helplessness? Well, scientists found out that the one variable which makes or breaks a kid is the perception of control. When a child facing adversity feels he or she had some level of control or influence on the outcome of whatever they were facing.

That's why the child could make a choice and develop grit when, on the contrary, the child felt he or she had no way to influence the situation they were in. Well, that they were just on the receiving end of bad luck. Well, that's where their young brains engraved that life is just what happens to them. And there's really no point in even trying to change that. Learned helplessness. You see how authority can easily backfire here. By being too strict, you can just break their spirit each time they come home with whatever accomplishment you say, 'why didn't you do better'?

Well, the message they're getting is 'whatever I do, it's never good enough'. So why even try? We need to be strict. We need to be demanding, but not too much. How does that work exactly? Well, being demanding is only one side of the story, the other one which is equally crucial to reach grit and not having authority backfire, is being supportive, demanding, yet supportive, supportive, yet demanding two sides of the same coin.

One shouldn't go without the other. Well, as my kids grow, I've become increasingly demanding. The support they always had. Me being demanding has stepped up. Gradually, you see, is the Prefrontal brain, which regulates impulse control and higher executive function. It is this Prefrontal brain which gradually comes online but is mostly absent in small kids. That's why most four years old or incapable of passing the marshmallow tests. They can't control their impulses, yet they go for instant gratification.

As always, there's absolutely no way we can hold them accountable for that. It's just it just wouldn't be fair. Why? Well, because our brains evolved for millions of years in a totally different context than the one, we're in today. Our brain evolved for immediate gratification. You see, in a world dominated by uncertainty, the smart choice was to go for the instant return and to not wait for days, months or even years to reap the fruits of our hard work 200,000 years ago. Every day could be our last one. So why resist temptation?

Another example of this is that our brains evolved for energy efficiency. They will always choose. The easy road to being lazy was a great survival strategy from an energy efficiency point of view. So now, look at your kids. They have the same brain between the ears, which is hardwired to do fun things, and avoid doing tedious stuff, especially if that demands effort and energy. And the only way to overcome that for themselves is to bring it up, to go against their instincts, the capacity of which lays in their still dormant prefrontal brain.

However, that changes and slowly but surely that Prefrontal brain is coming online. And as it does, I'm here reminding them, demanding them to take the hard road whenever I ask them to do something, being it for school or chores, and they're doing a lousy job. I used my favorite phrase, which is try hard. They hate it when I do that, but it's great. It's a very simple, straightforward message and has a huge advantage in that it puts them in control. It's their decision and they can influence it.

Try harder is what I expect from you. You're the one who can improve on the situation. It's in your hands. Now, remember the perception of control. Here it is. Try harder. Well, sometimes try harder. It comes down to trying things differently. But the message is the same. Keep trying. This is not good enough and you can change that. And then there's a second part, of course, demanding, yet supportive after saying try harder depending on the situation.

I will explain that I know they can do it better, that I believe in them, or sometimes I will explain the importance of grit. Oh, they know about grit. They know exactly how I think about that. But I talk with them. We discuss things. I will explain why I think it's important for them to do better. And I ask them their reasons for wanting, for example, to quit an activity. I usually try to convince them to continue some more. And we agree on a point of no return where they can stop if it really doesn't work out.

But when they do a lousy job and they know they didn't really try, they get no mercy from me. I will make it clear to them. We need to teach them to do the hard stuff, to take the difficult choice to overcome their brains predisposition for the easy and gratifying stuff, at one point it's no more fun and games. It's a gradual process, but they need to learn it. This is what they call tough love, tough and love. Both are important, just as demanding, yet supportive.

You remember when you were kids and your parents told you would thank me later? Well, this is it. You reached that point. You just turned into a younger version of your own mother or father, because grit is about exactly that. You're helping their future self to be a better version of themselves, and they will. Thank you. Later or not, you might need to help them connect the dots, in 30 years or so. Remember when I told you to clean your room and now you just won the Nobel Peace Prize? You're welcome. Sharpen your mind.

6.1 The perfect Parent

I remember vividly when I first held my baby girl in my arms, she was so small, she seemed so fragile, I could feel a terrifying sense of responsibility, overwhelming me. I felt like I would never be able to live up to this task that life had given me of raising a frail little creature into a beautiful, strong-willed and balanced young adult. I realized that there was so much that potentially could go wrong that for sure something would go wrong.

When I spoke about this fear of mine to an NBA colleague, he smiled and told me, that's OK. What do you mean? That's OK? I don't want my kid to be scared or traumatized. He looked at me and said, first of all, kids aren't that easily traumatized. Second, you can't protect them from everything. Even more so, you shouldn't protect them from everything as they need to learn how to deal with failure and pain. And last, but not least, you will make errors. As a parent, you will fail.

There will be moments when you are tired or stressed or just clumsy, and you will say or do things that you will regret afterwards. And guess what? It's no big deal. Nobody's perfect. No one. Not even you. And that's my message for you also. Nobody's perfect, not even you. The fact that you're taking this course means that you're taking the education of your kids seriously. Great. Now, all the best intentions in the world won't make you perfect either. And you know what they say about good intentions, right?

Parenting is difficult. It really is, there's no manual. All kids are different. What works with one won't work with another. It's often pure chaos and drama and tears. Recent research has shown that one of the populations most at risk to get a burnout are parents who stay at home to raise small kids. Not really. In some cases, it should almost be possible to sue those kids for emotional harassment I've seen in real situations.

You have no idea? Well, actually, you might if you've seen an episode of The Nanny, you know what I'm talking about. It's really hard. So don't put an extra burden on yourself by raising expectations to an unrealistic level. Remember this, you will make mistakes, and that's OK. Sharpen your mind.

6.2 You are raising your kid

As much as you might like to think that you are the sole guardian of the education of your children, the truth is you are only one of the many contributors to it. Kids are like sponges. They take in everything that flies by and information comes from all directions. The parents, of course, have a big chunk in it, but there is way more teachers at school, grandparents, uncles and aunts, brothers, sisters, friends at school or in the neighborhood, cousins, but also books, cartoons, television, music, bedtime stories, the Internet, social media games.

The list is almost endless, from the bus driver to fictional characters. They all leave their parents. Who will your child become? Yes, you are an important contributor to the education of your child. However, you are far from being the only one. So don't be too hard on yourself if things don't go as you planned or as you wished for. In a perfect world, raising a kid is a team effort.

However, that doesn't mean that you have no influence on that environment, on that team. On the contrary, you are one assembling the team. All decisions in that matter count from the neighborhood you live in, into the school you send them to, from the programs you let them watch, to your supervision of their social media use. There will always be elements in the team influencing your child in ways you would have preferred not to.

Whether that's it is good for your child to experience that. The world isn't a one-dimensional place, where there are other voices, other opinions, other ways of doing things that they can express parts of their personality in different ways with different people. If you make all the choices for them, how will they be able to learn to make their own?

It's only through these experiences, all of them, that they will be able to make up their own minds about what to do with their life, how to behave, what choices to make, who they want to hang out with, etc. And that, in the end, is probably the greatest education of all, giving them awareness. And that's activity, the strength of mind to make their own choices in life. Sharpen your mind.

6.3 You raised your kids in the same way... and yet...

There is always someone who explains how they raised their children the same way and how those two or three children are also different. Here's the thing, you like to think you raise your children in exactly the same way, unfortunately or fortunately, I should say, that's not what's happening. You see, a lot of studies have shown that the simple fact of having siblings, older or younger, does affect our personality. It's called the birth order effect. And it goes like this.

The first child will automatically get more attention from their parents. Not only is there no other child around to divert attention, but more importantly, parents will feel a strong urge to do everything as perfectly as possible. With a second or third child, the parent's attitude becomes much more relaxed as they have been there, done that, sense of having things under control, even without an iron grip on every single detail.

This leads to the first born often being more reliable, conscientious, structured, cautious, controlling and achievers. Common traits with firstborns are perfectionism and a competitive mindset. The middle transposition position is not easy. The first-born gets all the attention in the beginning and the last one grabbed the whole family's attention as this little baby is so cute. Basically, the middle child is left out.

So where does that lead to people pleasers that somewhat rebellious. They thrive on friendships, and they have a large social circle and are peacemakers. There is a variable here when the two children are not of the same gender. The oldest one is, let's say, a boy. The second one is still the first girl. So, she can end up with firstborn characteristics. For example, it's quite common to see in such a scenario. The second born becomes like a little mummy for the other kids, especially the younger ones.

Lazybones tend to be free spirited since their parents have been losing the reins more easily. So, the youngest one tends to be fun, loving, uncomplicated, manipulative, outgoing, attention seeker and self-centered. Now, with only children, we get another scenario. Without any siblings to compete with, the only child gets all his parents' attention not just for a short period of time like a firstborn, but forever.

This way, the only child ends up being some kind of extreme first born with falling consequences, they tend to be mature for their age, perfectionists, conscientious, diligent and leaders. Now, of course, plenty of exceptions do exist. We see that happening with blended families, for example, where birth order might reshuffle the cards or with twins who will never take the middle role. Large gaps between children also affect the role taken.

Adopted children are also likely to form an exception, as the age at which the adoption took place plays an important role. So, in conclusion, don't fool yourself. You're not raising your children in the same way, it's physically impossible because of the presence of the other children in your family. So, is that a bad thing? Of course not.

It helps create diversity. However, you as a parent shouldn't be surprised when your children turn out differently. On the one hand, there's the unpredictability of the natural shuffle of the genes. And on the other hand, you, despite all your efforts, are just predestined not to raise your children in the same way. Sharpen your mind.

6.4 Conclusion

Time to bring all this together, to bring it to a close you Super Kid: Super Smart. What have we learned? Well, we've seen how we have four different brain structures and our kids as well, obviously. And these brain structures tell us an important story about our needs and priorities in order to develop into healthy and balanced individuals. First, there was this primitive, primal, reptilian brain in charge of managing our vital physiological needs.

Now, here at this level, we focused on three things the importance of sleep. And I'm getting tired of repeating myself. But this one is so crucial, there is really no way to overstate this. Second, the importance of movement. They should play sports, get them to use that body as much as possible. Third is food. Food is more than fuel, it's also the building blocks for the growing brains.

So, help them develop a healthy diet. And it basically comes down to a Mediterranean diet, right? Fresh fruit and vegies, olive oil, fatty fish, etc. When we move to the limbic brain, we cover how we as human beings relate to others, how we form our identity in relation to the people around us. It impacts our self-confidence, how much we trust others, but also how much social exclusion hurts and thus why peer pressure works so well. And this is so much truer for our kids and teenagers.

With the new limbic brain, we enter the realm of rewards, punishments, expectations, but also the importance of grit and delayed gratification and of course, how to deal with screen time and with the prefrontal brain. We looked at how the brain deals with novelty and learning, but also how does brain structure is the last one to reach maturity and the far-reaching impact that has on our teenagers, especially regarding peer groups and risk taking.

And well, the careful observer will have noticed that the time of adolescence is a point where it all comes together. If you were able to find the crucial Paleo limbic balance towards assertiveness during that decade before adolescence, your teenager will be used to respecting rules on the one hand and have its own will to defy peer pressure. On the other hand, if you were able to, within that paleo limbic framework, give the necessary room for experiencing its new limbic natural talents.

Well, your teenager will have less reasons to experiment as he or she will already have discovered its uniqueness and strength. If you were able to withhold from too much cheering and encouraging the traits you wish to see your child develop, his motivation will also be much more embedded in his own intrinsic personality and less in what others think or expect from him, making him or her less of a crowd pleaser.

And of course, if you were able to prevent a small social trauma, even though some will have happened at school or elsewhere, your teenager won't be falling into the excesses caused by compensation mechanisms.

To summarize it all, I would bring it down to the following things, the main pillars for a healthy brain; sleep, movement and a healthy diet. Then there's grit, of course, you know, linked to delayed gratification and the growth mindset, which really is the cornerstone for success later in life. And then there are the three golden rules.

One, give your child a framework, a set of rules to within this framework, let him experiment and try things out with as little adult interfering as possible.

Let them find out for themselves what it is they like and dislike.

Three, avoid small social traumas, meaning public humiliations.

These three golden rules will help you get along way with your offspring. As in any relationship, there will be ups and downs. And if for one reason or another, tensions are rising, your relationship with your son or daughter, remember that the best way to deal with the primal brain is to take away the perceived danger. You are not the enemy. You are on their side. You're there to help. Now, once the primal brain is switched off, you can start a normal, rational conversation.

Well, rational. No, no, not really. Remember, our kids operate on the emotional level, not the rational one. And if we want our communication with them to be as effective as possible, we should put ourselves on their level, talk about emotions with them, acknowledge them, share our own emotions, and offer guidance.

And I can promise you one thing. Things will not go according to your plans; things are going to get messy. You will lose your nerves. You will yell, they will yell. There will be bad moments. You will want to see some reason in them. There will be bad moments. They will want to see some reasons. And you know, it's all the joys of parenting. And if one day you come home and you find, as I did, your daughter's hair all over the playroom, well, just take a deep breath and activate your Prefrontal brain by imagining yourself ten years from now. Looking back at this day. And another way is to remind yourself it could have been worse.

Neuro Geeks

6.5 Thank you

Congratulations! We've arrived at the end of this book.

I would like to thank you for having read it. Good luck with your children. I wish you tons of memorable, special moments together.

Because in the end, we are social beings. It's in our DNA. Why do you think we have such a sophisticated speaking capacity?

www.ingramcontent.com/pod-product-compliance
Lightning Source LLC
Chambersburg PA
CBHW021616270326
41931CB00008B/727